Clinician's Illustrated Dictionary of HYPERTENSION A-F

Presented as a service to cardiovascular medicine by
Servier Laboratories Limited

Clinician's Illustrated Dictionary of HYPERTENSION A-F

Gordon W Herd

MRC Blood Pressure Unit, Western Infirmary, Glasgow

Stephen G Ball

Professor of Cardiovascular Studies, University of Leeds

John D Swales

Professor of Medicine, University of Leicester

science press

© Copyright 1988 by Science Press Limited
Phillipp House
20 Chancellor's Street
Hammersmith Riverside
London W6 9RL, UK

British Library Cataloguing in Publication Data

1.   Hypertension
I   Herd, Gordon W   II Ball, Stephen G
III   Swales, John D
616.1'32 RC685-H8

ISBN 1-870026-25-X

Designer: Medilink Design, London
Illustrator: Maurizia Merati

Printed and bound in Italy by Imago Publishing Limited.

Introduction

The Clinician's Illustrated Dictionary of Hypertension is a comprehensive work of reference which aims to provide authoritative definitions and explanations of terms and concepts currently used in clinical hypertension. The enormous expansion in our knowledge of high blood pressure has led to new means of diagnosis and treatment which have revolutionized the outlook of the individual patient.

Many disciplines have contributed to this new understanding including biochemistry, physiology, pharmacology and epidemiology. Each of these has to some extent developed its own language: this frequently confuses the clinician and the non-medically qualified staff who help him.

A world-wide panel of experts has therefore been gathered to provide authoritative definitions and explanations.

Important topics are covered by means of larger signed entries by acknowledged international authorities.

Duplication has been avoided by an extensive cross-referencing system. Where important concepts or diseases are associated with particular individuals, brief biographical information has been included. We trust that this dictionary will be of value to practitioners at all stages of their career as well as their staff.

John D Swales
Stephen G Ball
Gordon W Herd

December 1987

A

Accelerated hypertension
A term used by some to denote severe hypertension with retinal haemorrhages and exudates, but without papilloedema. Recent studies suggest that cases with and without papilloedema have the same prognosis.Many people consider that the terms accelerated and malignant hypertension should embrace all hypertensive patients with bilateral haemorrhages and exudates related to hypertension, irrespective of the presence or absence of papilloedema. See also *Hypertensive retinopathy: Malignant phase hypertension*

ACE
see *Angiotensin I converting enzyme*

Acebutalol
A beta-adrenergic antagonist. See also *Beta-adrenergic receptor blocking drugs*

Acetylator status
The genetically determined difference in the ability to acetylate certain drugs: for instance, slow acetylators of hydralazine are more likely to develop drug-induced systemic lupus erythematosus. See also *Drug-induced lupus*

Acetylcholine (ACh)
An important neurotransmitter present in postganglionic parasympathetic, preganglionic autonomic, somatic motor, and some central nervous system neurones.
Acetylcholine released from these neurones binds to cholinergic receptors. After the neurotransmitter has served its function it is hydrolyzed by acetylcholinesterase.
Acetylcholine given by intravenous infusion in man at around 40 mg/min causes vasodilatation and lowering of the blood pressure, but the negative inotropic and chronotropic effects of the agent

are not seen due to rapid enzymatic hydrolysis. At larger doses hypotension is accompanied by bradycardia.
Vasodilatation induced by acetylcholine in practically all vascular beds is caused by binding of the neurotransmitter to vascular muscarinic receptors despite the lack of a cholinergic nerve supply to most blood vessels. These muscarinic receptors involved appear to be in the vascular endothelial cells. A vasorelaxant substance released from these cells may act on the vascular smooth muscle cells.
Studies using animal models suggest that alterations in central nervous system cholinergic transmission are associated with hypertension, for example see, *Hemicholinium-3*

Acetylcholinesterase (AChE)
An enzyme which catalyzes the hydrolysis of the neurotransmitter acetylcholine and is therefore a major determinant of the inactivation of the neurotransmitter after release. It is found in nervous tissue and in red blood cells. See also *Acetylcholine: Cholinesterase*

Acromegalogigantism
Gigantism and acromegaly caused by excessive secretion of growth hormone beginning before puberty and persisting into adult life.

Acromegaloidism
A condition with features similar to acromegaly but without growth hormone excess.

Acromegaly
A disease caused by excessive secretion of growth hormone after puberty by an adenoma or occasionally hyperplasia of the acidophil cells of the anterior pituitary gland.
Clinical features include enlargement of the hands, feet and jaw, with a character-istic facial appearance (Figure 1).
Acromegaly may cause headache, fatigue, arthropathy (50%),

Acromegaly

carpal tunnel syndrome, sexual dysfunction, congestive cardiac failure and hypertension (30-40%). The mechanism of the hypertension is unclear. Diagnosis can usually be made by demonstrating failure of suppression of growth hormone during an oral glucose tolerance test.
A large adenoma may cause enlargement of the sella turcica visible on a lateral skull x-ray. Smaller adenomas may be demonstrated by pituitary computed tomography.
Treatment is primarily by surgical removal of the tumour, but bromocriptine is also used.
Cure of growth hormone excess may improve blood pressure in hypertensive patients with acromegaly.

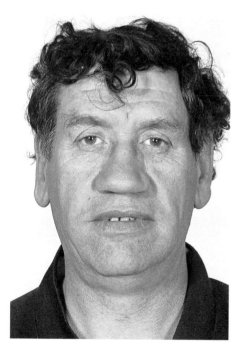

Figure 1 Acromegaly. Acromegalic facies

ACTH (adrenocorticotrophic hormone)
(*also known as* Adrenocorticotrophin: Corticotrophin) A polypeptide with 39 amino acid residues secreted by the anterior pituitary gland and acting mainly on the adrenal cortex, stimulating its growth and the secretion of cortico-steroids, chiefly cortisol.
ACTH or related peptides may also be produced by tumours of the lung, thymus, pancreatic islet cells and others in the ectopic ACTH syndrome. See also *Cortisol: Cushing's disease: Cushing's syndrome: Pro-opiomelanocortin*

ACTH-dependent hyperaldosteronism
see *Dexamethasone-suppressible aldosteronism*

ACTH-produced hypertension
The infusion of ACTH may induce hypertension in some species. Hypertension can arise from oversecretion of ACTH from hypothalamic-pituitary dysfunction or more rarely from ectopic ACTH from various tumours. See also *Cushing's syndrome*

Actin
A major protein forming the thin filament of skeletal and cardiac muscle. Contraction occurs when thin and thick filaments slide past one another without change in length of the filaments themselves. Smooth muscle cells contain a less ordered pattern of these filaments. See also *Actin-myosin interaction: Myosin: Vascular smooth muscle*

Actin-myosin interaction
Myosin molecules form the thick filaments of the sarcomere. These use the energy of ATP hydrolysis to move along thin filaments. The two filaments thus 'slide' past one another and muscle contracts. The interaction occurs in both smooth and skeletal muscle but there are important differences, in particular, latch formation allows sustained contraction at low energy cost in smooth muscle. See also *Actin: Myosin: Sarcomere: Vascular smooth muscle*

Active transport
The movement of ions or molecules across a cell membrane from a region of low to high concentration at the expense of energy provided by cellular chemical reactions.

Actomyosin
This is a complex formed between the proteins actin and myosin in muscle. See also *Actin: Actin-myosin interaction: Myosin*

Actomyosin ATPase activity
The ability of the actomyosin complex to catalyze the hydrolysis of adenosine triphosphate, producing adenosine diphosphate, and to release energy important for muscle contraction. See also *Actin: Myosin*

Addison's disease
(Thomas Addison, English physician, 1793-1860)
Primary adrenal failure most commonly caused by either autoimmune disease or tuberculosis of the adrenals. Common clinical features include pigmentation, lassitude, weight loss, nausea, abdominal pain, and postural hypotension.
A routine biochemical screen may reveal the combination of low serum sodium, high serum potassium and high serum urea concentrations but this is unusual except with impending crisis.
Diagnosis can usually be made by failure of the plasma cortisol to rise appropriately in a Synacthen test. In the autoimmune type, adrenal autoantibodies are usually present and other autoimmune disease may also be present or develop, for example insulin-dependent diabetes mellitus. Patients are treated with cortisol replacement (20-30 mg daily) and may also require mineralocorticoid replacement in the form of fludrocortisone. Stress, such as major surgery, will require an increase in the dosage of cortisol. See also *Adrenal glands*

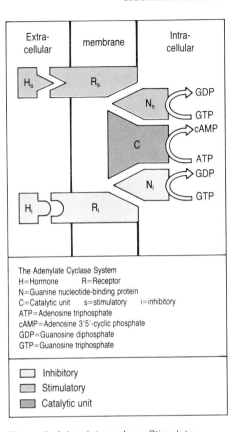

The Adenylate Cyclase System
H=Hormone   R=Receptor
N=Guanine nucleotide-binding protein
C=Catalytic unit   s=stimulatory   i=inhibitory
ATP=Adenosine triphosphate
cAMP=Adenosine 3'5'-cyclic phosphate
GDP=Guanosine diphosphate
GTP=Guanosine triphosphate

☐ Inhibitory
☐ Stimulatory
▨ Catalytic unit

Figure 2 Adenylate cyclase. Stimulatory agonist H_s binds to the high affinity RN complex to form the HRN ternary complex. GTP binds to HRN complex, disassociates it to the lower affinity form and simultaneously activates N. The activated N-GTP complex then activates the catalytic unit. This catalyzes the formation of adenosine 3'5'-cyclic phosphate (cAMP) which then activates cAMP-dependent protein kinase. The process is terminated by GTPase activity on N which catalyzes hydrolysis of GTP, de-activating the system. Since agonists, but not antagonists, bind to RN with high affinity, only the former favour formation of the ternary complex. In the case of inhibitory agonists (Hi), the activated N-GTP complex deactivates the catalytic unit following Hi binding

3

Adenosine

Adenosine
The nucleoside adenine-D-ribose.

Adenosine 3′:5′-cyclic phosphate (cAMP)
A cyclic nucleotide which acts as the 'second messenger' for several important hormones including catecholamines, glucagon and ACTH.
The intracellular effects of cAMP are mediated by cAMP-dependent protein kinase. Reaction with cAMP activates the latter enzyme which then phosphorylates a variety of proteins, for instance enzymes, either activating or deactivating them in the process. See also *Adenylate cyclase*

Adenylate cyclase
A membrane-bound enzyme which catalyzes the conversion of adenosine triphosphate to adenosine 3′:5′-cyclic phosphate. It is activated or inhibited when certain hormones bind to their receptors and interact with guanine nucleotide binding proteins (Figure 2).

ADH
see *Antidiuretic hormone*

Adrenal adenomas
Benign neoplasms of the adrenal cortex which may secrete aldosterone, producing primary aldosteronism resulting in Conn's syndrome, or cortisol, producing Cushing's syndrome.
Adrenal adenomas may also cause virilization or feminization. Non-functioning adrenocortical adenomas may not, in fact, be true neoplasms and are termed adrenal nodules by some. (Figure 3) See also *Conn's syndrome; Cushing's disease*

Adrenal angiotensin receptors
see *Angiotensin receptors*

Adrenal computed tomography (adrenal CT scanning)
Aldosterone-secreting adenomas are frequently small but CT scanning usually

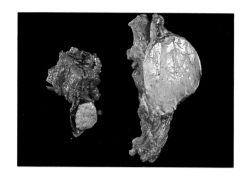

Figure 3 Adrenal adenoma. Adrenal adenoma and nodule: Adrenal glands from a patient who had an aldosterone-secreting adenoma on the left, and a larger nodule (non-functioning adenoma) in the right adrenal gland

detects tumours greater than 1 cm diameter (Figure 4).
Phaeochromocytomas in the adrenal are often larger at presentation and are readily detected but the major limitation of CT scanning for phaeochromocytomas is in the detection of extra-adrenal lesions, particularly when multiple. See also *Computed tomography*

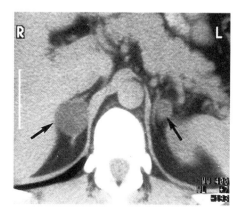

Figure 4 Adrenal computed tomography. Adrenal CT scan from the patient whose adrenal glands are illustrated in Figure 3. The bilateral masses are clearly shown (arrowed)

Adrenal cortex

The outer part of the adrenal gland, which consists of three major histologically distinct regions within a fibrous capsule. Beneath the capsule is the zona glomerulosa (zg), inside is the widest region, the zona fasciculata (zf), and next to the medulla is the inner zona reticularis (zr) where glucocorticoids, androgens and progestogens are produced. Aldosterone is formed in the zg only. Cortisol is formed largely in the inner zones, mainly the zf. (Figure 5)

Adrenal glands

(*also known as* Suprarenal glands) These two glands are each situated at the cranial pole of the corresponding kidney at about the level of the first lumbar vertebra. The right gland is pyramidal. The left gland is semilunar, and slightly larger than the right.

The arterial supply of the glands is somewhat variable. The venous drainage (Figure 6) is clinically important due to the use of adrenal venous sampling, particularly in the diagnosis of Conn's

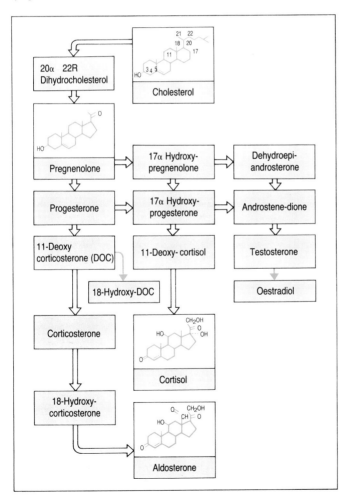

Figure 5 Adrenal cortex. Adrenocortical hormone synthesis

Adrenal glands

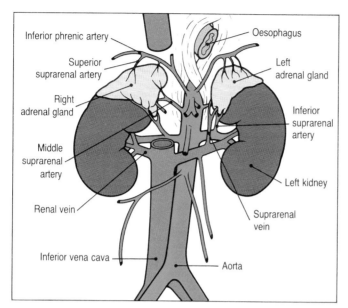

Inferior phrenic artery

Superior suprarenal artery

Right adrenal gland

Middle suprarenal artery

Renal vein

Inferior vena cava

Oesophagus

Left adrenal gland

Inferior suprarenal artery

Left kidney

Suprarenal vein

Aorta

Figure 6 Adrenal glands. The adrenal glands and their blood supply. The terms 'adrenal' and 'suprarenal' are synonymous. The right suprarenal vein drains into the inferior vena cava, the left drains into the left renal vein

syndrome. The outer part of each gland (cortex) secretes steroid hormones, while the inner part (medulla) secretes catecholamines (mainly adrenaline in humans). See also *Adrenal venous sampling*

Adrenal hyperplasia
The term hyperplasia implies an abnormal increase in the number of cells in a given gland or tissue.
Hyperplasia may occur in both the cortex and the medulla but the term is more commonly applied to disorders of the cortex.
Congenital adrenal hyperplasia (CAH) is a group of congenital disorders of adrenocortical steroid-synthesizing enzymes which may present at different times from the neonatal period to adult life. 11-β-hydroxylase and 17-α-hydroxylase deficiencies cause hypertension and hypokalaemia with suppressed renin but normal plasma aldosterone concentrations.
Bilateral micronodular hyperplasia of the zona glomerulosa is associated with

hypertension and hypokalaemia but with high circulating concentrations of aldosterone in an older age group (idiopathic or non-tumorous aldosteronism).
Hyperplasia of the medulla is said to occur in the early stages of phaeochromocytoma formation in patients with multiple endocrine neoplasia syndromes. See also *Hyperplasia: Idiopathic aldosteronism*

Adrenal medulla
The inner part of adrenal gland made up of chromaffin cells (derived from neural crest ectoderm) which form catecholamines, predominantly adrenaline.

Adrenal nodules
These nodules are localized growths of adrenocortical cells which some regard as variations of adrenal structure associated with ageing rather than being true neoplasms. They may be the same as the masses described as non-functioning adrenal adenomas. The nodules are frequent incidental autopsy findings and

may also occur in association with a variety of adrenal disorders including primary aldosteronism due to an aldosteronoma. They may also be found incidentally during abdominal computed tomography.

Adrenal scintigraphy
This imaging technique visualizes the adrenals because of the cortical uptake of radioactively-labelled cholesterol derivatives (Figure 7).
The radionuclide iodo-benzyl guanidine is used to demonstrate tumours of the medulla. See also *MIBG scanning*

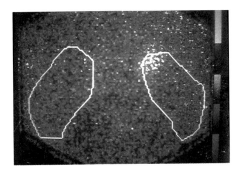

Figure 7 Adrenal scintigraphy. Adrenal scintigraphic scan showing uptake of the radionuclide by a right-sided adrenal adenoma. Renal outlines are also shown

Adrenal ultrasonography
(*also known as* Adrenal ultrasound scanning) This examination of the adrenal glands using ultrasound techniques is non-invasive, but technically demanding. It is useful for identifying large aldosterone-producing adenomas, but not the more common smaller tumours. Many phaeochromocytomas are large at presentation and ultrasound examination may readily detect tumours as small as 3 cm.

Adrenal venography
A technique for demonstrating the vasculature of the adrenals by injecting contrast medium into the adrenal veins.

Used to outline, for example, adrenocortical adenomas (Figure 8). This technique carries a small risk of adrenal infarction.

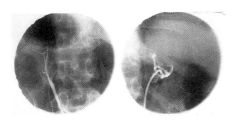

Figure 8 Adrenal venogram. Adrenal venogram showing the vessels outlining a right-sided adrenal adenoma (right of picture). The patient's left adrenal gland is normal (left of picture)

Adrenal venous sampling
Measurement of aldosterone in adrenal venous plasma is still the most reliable method of determining the site of an aldosterone-producing adenoma (Figure 9) or distinguishing primary aldosteronism due to a tumour from idiopathic aldosteronism. It can be technically difficult, however, and carries a small risk of adrenal infarction.

Adrenal zona glomerulosa (fasciculata, reticularis)
see *Adrenal cortex*

Adrenalectomy
The surgical removal of adrenal glands. Adrenalectomy is usually the treatment recommended in patients with primary aldosteronism associated with an aldosterone-secreting adenoma (Conn's syndrome). The operation is more likely to cure the hypertension if there has been a good blood pressure response to preoperative spironolactone or amiloride. Bilateral adrenalectomy may be required in patients with multiple endocrine neoplasia who have bilateral adrenomedullary hyperplasia or phaeochromocytoma.

Adrenaline

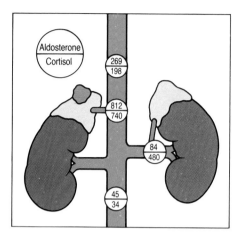

Figure 9 Adrenal venous sampling. Adrenal venous sampling with measurements of plasma aldosterone and cortisol concentration in a patient with a right-sided aldosterone-secreting adrenal adenoma. Concentrations are in picomoles per litre, and the figures for aldosterone can be seen to be much higher in the right adrenal vein compared with the left. Cortisol is also measured to confirm that the catheters were correctly positioned

Adrenaline

(*also known as* Epinephrine)
Catecholamine synthesized in the adrenal medulla (Figure 10a) and secreted with smaller amounts of noradrenaline. (This is the case in dogs and humans. In cats and some other species noradrenaline is the main hormone secreted by the adrenal medulla.)
Adrenaline also functions as a neurotransmitter in the central nervous system. The hormone has numerous effects resulting from stimulation of both alpha- and beta-adrenergic receptors. Its cardiovascular effects are complex, and depend to some degree on the mode and duration of administration. A rapid intravenous bolus causes a rise in blood pressure which rapidly reaches a peak proportional to the dose administered. As systolic pressure rises more than diastolic pressure, mean pressure also increases. As the response wears off, mean arterial pressure becomes subnormal before returning to the control level. The increased pressure results from a positive inotropic effect, a positive chronotropic effect, and, most importantly, vasoconstriction in many vascular beds. Bradycardia may be found at the peak of the blood pressure response due to compensatory vagal stimulation.

Prolonged intravenous infusion
Adrenaline has somewhat different effects when given by prolonged intravenous infusion. Systolic pressure rises moderately due to the positive inotropic and chronotropic effects, and cardiac output increases. However, diastolic pressure usually falls due to the decreased peripheral resistance resulting from stimulation of vascular beta$_2$-receptors in skeletal muscle and liver (which tends to overcome vasoconstriction produced elsewhere). These effects contrast with those of slow intravenous infusion of noradrenaline (Figure 10b). Since adrenaline causes little increase in mean arterial pressure, there are no compensatory effects such as increased vagal tone.

Vascular effects
Adrenaline acts principally on the smaller arterioles, and it has different effects on different vascular beds. In the skin, the hormone causes vasoconstriction and results in pallor. In muscle, adrenaline tends to cause increased blood flow partly due to beta$_2$ stimulation. Hepatic blood flow is also increased. Renal blood flow is reduced by doses of adrenaline which have little effect on mean arterial pressure. Coronary blood flow is increased. Apart from its effects on the blood supply of the kidney, adrenaline also stimulates secretion of renin by its effect on the beta$_1$-receptors of the juxtaglomerular

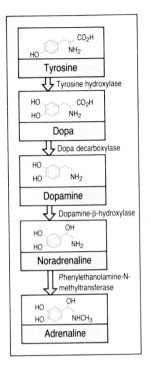

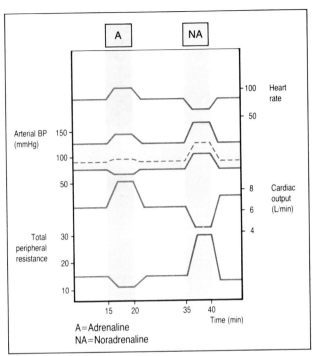

Figure 10(a) Adrenaline. Adrenaline synthesis

Figure 10(b) Adrenaline. Effect of slow intravenous infusion of adrenaline and noradrenaline

apparatus. The hormone also has complex metabolic effects, and effects on the central nervous, respiratory and other systems.

'Fight or flight'

Increased secretion of adrenaline by the adrenal medulla is part of the reaction which prepares an individual for 'fight or flight'. However, experimental work suggests that the action of secreted catecholamines on the vascular system is of little significance compared with the effects of noradrenergic nerve discharges. The metabolic effects of circulating catecholamines are probably more important in this context. See also *Catecholamines and hypertension: Noradrenaline: Phaeochromocytoma*

Adrenalitis

Inflammation of the adrenal glands.

Adrenergic

Stimulated by, employing, or secreting adrenaline (strictly) or other catecholamines. Used synonymously with noradrenergic.

Adrenergic neurone blocking agents

Drugs which probably impair transmitter release from the adrenergic postganglionic sympathetic neurone.

Members of this group include guanethidine, debrisoquine, bethanidine and bretylium tosylate. Postural hypotension, dry mouth and failure of ejaculation are common side-effects. Now

Adrenergic neurone blocking agents

little used in clinical practice in many countries.

Adrenergic receptor blocking drugs (adrenergic antagonists)

Drugs which act as antagonists at adrenergic receptors. Many such agents, acting at beta- and alpha-adrenergic receptors, have hypotensive effects.

Adrenergic receptors (adrenoceptors)

Membrane-bound proteins to which catecholamines bind with high affinity and produce their effects. They are divided into beta$_1$ and beta$_2$ plus alpha$_1$ and alpha$_2$ subtypes (Table 1). See also *Alpha-adrenergic receptors: Beta-adrenergic receptors*

Adrenoceptors

see *Adrenergic receptors*

Adrenochrome

Oxidation product of adrenaline which has been used as an experimental psychomimetic.

Adrenocortical carcinoma

A malignant tumour of the adrenal cortex. These tumours may secrete cortisol or androgens, but rarely oestrogens or aldosterone. See also *Adrenal cortex: Cushing's syndrome*

Adrenocorticotrophic hormone: Adrenocorticotrophin

Synonyms for ACTH.

Table 1 Adrenergic receptors

	$\alpha 1$	$\alpha 2$	$\beta 1$	$\beta 2$
Agonist potency	A ≥ NA >> PE >> I	A ≥ NA >> PE >> I	I > A ≥ NA > PE	I > A >> NA > PE
Specific antagonists	Prazosin	Yohimbine rauwolscine	Atenolol metoprolol	ICI 118,551
Responses	Smooth muscle contraction in blood vessels and genitourinary tract	Smooth muscle relaxation in gastrointestinal tract. Smooth muscle contraction in selected vascular beds.	Increased rate and force of cardiac contraction	Smooth muscle relaxation in bronchi, blood vessels, genitourinary and gastrointestinal tracts
	Activation of glycogenolysis (rat liver)	Inhibition of NA release from sympathetic nerve terminals	Stimulation of lipolysis	Facilitation of NA release
		Inhibition of lipolysis in adipocytes	Stimulation of renin release by juxtaglomerular cells	Increased hepatic glycogenolysis and gluconeogenesis
		Platelet aggregation		Increased muscular glycogenolysis
		Inhibition of renin release from juxtaglomerular cells of kidney		
		Inhibition of insulin release by pancreatic cells		Increased insulin and glucagon secretion by pancreatic cells
Location	Post synaptic	Presynaptic, postsynaptic and non-synaptic eg platelets	Post synaptic	Presynaptic, postsynaptic and non-synaptic eg lymphocytes, polymorphs
Mechanism	Alterations of cellular calcium ion fluxes	Inhibition of adenylate cyclase	Stimulation of adenylate cyclase	Stimulation of adenylate cyclase

A = Adrenaline ; NA = Noradrenaline ; PE = Phenylephrine ; I = Isoprenaline

Adrenolutin
Metabolite of adrenaline.

Adrenolytic
Inhibiting the action of adrenergic
neurones or impairing the response
to adrenaline.

Adrenopause
Cessation of function of the adrenal
glands.

Adrenoprival
Pertaining to deprivation of adrenal
function or of the adrenal glands.

Adrenostatic
Diminishing the function of the adrenal
glands.

Adventitia (tunica adventitia)
Layer of loose connective tissue forming
the outermost covering of an organ or
vessel. See also *Arterial wall*

Afflux
Flow of a liquid or blood to a part.

Age
Frequency of arterial hypertension
increases with age (Table 2) except in
certain populations, for example Cuna

and Yanamamo Indians, Congo pygmies,
Kalahari bushmen, the rural Zulu and the
aborigines of Australia. Such populations
are generally tribal and live a fairly
'primitive' life. Migration of, for example,
rural Zulus to an urban environment, is
associated with a rise in blood pressure
with age. In Western populations where
blood pressure does rise with age, it is not
clear whether the change occurs generally
or if it is limited only to a hypertensive
fraction of the population. Certainly the
age of the patient needs to be considered
in the decision as to what level of blood
pressure requires treatment. See also
*Children and hypertension: Elderly and
hypertension: European Working Party
on Hypertension in the Elderly Study: Low
sodium, low blood pressure populations*

Agonist
Substance which has affinity for a given
receptor and binding of which stimulates
a physiological response. See also
Antagonist: Receptors

Albumin (albumen)
An important protein found in the blood.
Many drugs, for instance propranolol, bind
reversibly to it. If two or more drugs which
bind to albumin are being used one drug
may displace the other from the binding

| Table 2 Age: prevalence of hypertension with increasing age ||||||
| Age (y) | Lower Range* (%) || Higher Range** (%) || Total (%) ||
	Men	Women	Men	Women	Men	Women
25-34	6.6	1.7	0.9	0.5	7.5	2.2
35-44	10.9	3.9	3.1	2.7	14.0	6.6
45-54	15.7	10.1	6.9	3.8	22.6	13.9
55-64	18.4	21.4	6.8	6.2	25.2	27.6
65-74	25.9	29.5	4.9	5.4	30.8	34.9

Hypertension here defined as Systolic ≥160 and/or Diastolic ≥95mmHg.
*Diastolic 95-104 mmHg.
**Diastolic ≥105 mmHg.

sites on albumin. This would produce a higher free concentration of the displaced drug with potentially toxic effect since only the unbound drug is active.

Alcohol (special contribution from Dr D J. Stott, Gartnavel General Hospital, Glasgow, Scotland)
In general, regular alcohol consumption raises blood pressure.
Most epidemiological studies show that systolic pressure rises by 1mmHg for each 10 grams of alcohol (equivalent to half pint of beer or 1/5 gill spirits) consumed per day. Diastolic pressure rises by a lesser amount.
Controversy, however, still exists over the shape of the regression line relating blood pressure to alcohol intake. In some studies, this is J-shaped, that is, modest alcohol ingestion is associated with a lower blood pressure than is total abstinence. Increases in pressure are seen within 3-4 days of starting drinking. Moderation of alcohol intake results in a gradual reduction of blood pressure, and should be advised in all hypertensive patients who drink regularly. The mechanisms by which chronic alcohol ingestion raises blood pressure remain uncertain.
Acute alcohol ingestion has only minor effects on blood pressure in healthy subjects. There is an early rise in the systolic pressure, probably related more to the intake of calories and the associated metabolic effects than the alcohol itself. Subsequently, during the period of intoxication, blood pressure tends to be reduced due to a combination of decreased myocardial contractility, vasodilatation, and decreased circulating plasma volume secondary to inhibition of antidiuretic hormone release and the consequent water diuresis. A marked reflex tachycardia occurs which minimizes the reduction in blood pressure.
There are no significant alterations in blood pressure during the hangover period after a single dose of alcohol. These effects should be distinguished from those suffered by alcoholics who during true withdrawal from alcohol often become hypertensive probably from activation of the sympathetic nervous system, and perhaps increased cortisol production. This is temporary. Blood pressure settles as symptoms of tremor, sweating and tachycardia subside.

Aldosterone
Main human mineralocorticoid hormone. A steroid secreted from the zona glomerulosa of the adrenal cortex in response to angiotensin II, alteration in serum potassium concentration, and ACTH. Secretion is inhibited by atrial natriuretic peptide.

Aldosterone antagonists
Drugs, for example, spironolactone, which compete with aldosterone for binding to its receptor. Binding of spironolactone to the receptor protein prevents the latter from assuming the active conformation. Aldosterone antagonists act as potassium-sparing diuretics by reducing sodium reabsorption and potassium secretion in the distal convoluted tubules of the kidney.
See also *Mineralocorticoid receptors*

Aldosteronism
(*also known as* Hyperaldosteronism)
Hypersecretion of aldosterone which may be primary (in which case plasma renin activity is low) or secondary.
Primary aldosteronism is usually caused by an adrenal adenoma (aldosteronoma) or by bilateral adrenal hyperplasia. Low-renin aldosteronism is rarely associated with adrenal carcinomas, and very rarely with ovarian tumours.
Secondary aldosteronism is found under conditions in which renin secretion is stimulated, for example, renal artery stenosis or nephrotic syndrome with decreased effective blood volume.

Aldosteronism, bilateral
see *Bilateral aldosteronism*

Aldosteronism, dexamethasone-suppressible
see *Dexamethasone-suppressible aldosteronism*

Aldosteronoma
Aldosterone-producing adrenocortical adenoma

Alkyl ether analogues of phosphatidylcholine
see *Antihypertensive polar renomedullary lipid*

Alpha-adrenergic receptors
Studies of the relative potencies of various agonists acting at adrenergic receptors allow these receptors to be divided into alpha- and beta-adrenergic receptors. Alpha-receptors have subsequently been subdivided into alpha$_1$-receptors and alpha$_2$-receptors. Alpha$_1$-receptors predominate at the postsynaptic sites on smooth muscle and glandular cells. Alpha$_2$-receptors are located largely on presynaptic nerve terminals, where stimulation of these receptors causes inhibition of release of neurotransmitters including noradrenaline and acetylcholine. There is evidence also, however, for postsynaptic and nonsynaptic alpha$_2$-receptors. Some of the central nervous system postsynaptic alpha-adrenergic receptors are alpha$_2$-receptors (alpha$_2$-agonist drugs). Specific antagonists are available for both alpha-adrenergic receptor sub-types (see Table 1). Binding of an agonist to an alpha$_2$-receptor causes inhibition of adenylate cyclase, whereas the function of alpha$_1$-receptors is mediated by changes in intracellular calcium.

Alpha-adrenergic receptor blocking drugs
Antagonism at alpha-adrenergic receptors. *Prazosin* binds reversibly specifically to alpha$_1$-receptors lowering vascular tone on both the arterial and venous sides of the circulation. It is an effective antihypertensive agent.
Phentolamine also binds reversibly to alpha$_1$-receptors, but in addition blocks alpha$_2$-receptors. This latter effect on the presynaptic alpha$_2$-receptors enhances the release of noradrenaline from nerve endings, and may contribute to the tendency for phentolamine to cause cardiac arrhythmias. Phentolamine has been used in tests for diagnosing phaeochromocytoma, and also in the treatment of crises in this condition. *Phenoxybenzamine* causes blockade of both alpha$_1$- and alpha$_2$-receptors by reacting irreversibly (forming a covalent bond) with these receptors. Blockade with this drug develops relatively slowly and persists for some time after the drug is discontinued. Phenoxybenzamine is used mainly in the preoperative management of phaeochromocytoma, or for continued control of blood pressure in patients with inoperable tumours. Side-effects, including reflex tachycardia, have led to little use of phentolamine and phenoxybenzamine except in the treatment of phaeo-chromocytoma.

Alpha$_2$-agonist drugs
Drugs which stimulate alpha$_2$-receptors. Clonidine lowers blood pressure by stimulating central alpha$_2$-receptors and reducing sympathetic outflow. The anatomical site of action is unclear. Stimulation of presynaptic alpha$_2$-receptors may be less significant in its action than stimulation of postsynaptic alpha$_2$-receptors in the brain stem. See also *Clonidine: Clonidine suppression test*

Alpha-methyldopa
A centrally acting antihypertensive drug which still has a role in management if other drugs are contraindicated or not tolerated.
The main side-effects of alpha-methyldopa are sedation, postural hypotension, dry mouth and headache. Rarer toxic effects include haemolytic anaemia, thrombocyto-penia, leucopenia, hepatitis and lupus-

13

Alpha-methyldopa

like syndrome. See also
Centrally acting antihypertensive drugs

Alpha-methyltyrosine
Synonym for metyrosine.

Alphalytic
Acting as an antagonist at an alpha-adrenergic receptor.

Alphamimetic
Stimulating the alpha-adrenergic receptors of the sympathetic nervous system.

Alprenolol
Beta-adrenergic antagonist. See also *Beta-adrenergic receptor blocking drugs*

Alprostadil
Prostaglandin E_1. A prostaglandin with vasodilator properties.

Amaurosis fugax
Fleeting loss of vision in one eye caused by embolism into a retinal artery from a proximal site of atherosclerosis. See also *Transient ischaemic attacks*

Ambulatory blood pressure monitoring
(special contribution from Dr H.R. Brunner, Département de Médecine, Centre Hospitalier Universitaire Vaudois, Lausanne, Switzerland)
Portable devices exist which make it possible to record the blood pressure for up to 24 hours in ambulatory subjects. Some devices monitor pressure via an intra-arterial catheter connected to a pressure transducer and a recorder. They have the advantage of measuring blood pressure beat to beat during 24 hours, that is, waking and sleeping periods but their disadvantage is the requirement of an intra-arterial catheter.
Most other machines measure blood pressure non-invasively using the usual blood pressure measuring cuff on the arm, which is inflated sporadically (see *Korotkoff's sounds: Measurement of blood pressure*).

Automatic instruments inflate the cuff with a pump at predetermined intervals ranging usually from 10 to 30 minutes. Semi-automatic devices require that the patient himself inflates the cuff to a predetermined pressure which then activates the measuring procedure. While the automatic machines will record blood pressure during waking and sleeping hours, the semi-automatic recorders provide only measurements during day-time.
The advantage of both types is their non-invasive approach to blood pressure recording, their disadvantage is the sporadic nature of the blood pressure measurements. However, a recent comparative study has established quite clearly that the average of blood pressures measured at intervals of up to 30 minutes during 24 hours represents quite well the average of all blood pressures determined invasively during the same periods. Since with the non-invasive approach no beat to beat analysis of blood pressure is possible, the variability of blood pressure, which might represent an important factor in the pathogenesis of arterial lesions, cannot be assessed (see *Labile hypertension*). New devices presently under development which measure arteriolar blood pressure non-invasively via a cuff around the finger are very attractive. They do allow beat to beat analysis of blood pressure and if they can be miniaturized to become portable, they could potentially combine all the advantages of the available non-invasive monitors.
Why is there a need for ambulatory blood pressure monitoring?
As blood pressure is extremely variable depending on physical activity, posture, emotional status and many other factors, it does not seem intellectually satisfactory to base diagnostic and therapeutic decisions on one or two measurements obtained by the physician at intervals of several weeks. In other words, more measurements provide a statistically more solid basis from which to draw any

conclusions. As already mentioned, blood pressure variability and the shape of the daily blood pressure profile may represent independent factors playing an active role in the pathogenesis of atherosclerosis. It is therefore necessary to learn more about these parameters.

Probably the most important however is the phenomenon known as *'white coat syndrome'*. It has been known for a long time that hypertensive patients, when they measure their own blood pressure, often find considerably lower levels than their physician. This discrepancy has been confirmed many times using ambulatory blood pressure monitoring. Averaging all measurements recorded during the day-time in the ambulatory state away from the physician's office provides values in 70% to 80% of all normotensive and hypertensive patients which are clearly lower than those obtained by the physician in his office. If the differences were consistent, this would not present a major problem. However, experience has shown that in the individual patient, the difference between office measurement and ambulatory recording is completely unpredictable. In treated hypertensive patients it can range from −75 to +10 mmHg for systolic blood pressure with only slightly smaller discrepancies for diastolic blood pressure. Thus, if one wants to know in a given individual patient the blood pressure prevailing when he is pursuing his usual activities, ambulatory blood pressure monitoring rather than the measurement in the physician's office is more likely to provide the correct answer. While this difference may be smaller when the blood pressure is measured by a nurse rather than the physician, it still remains considerable. Measurements that come closest to ambulatory monitoring are those obtained by the patient himself.

What has been learned so far from ambulatory blood pressure monitoring, and what do we expect from the future?
The main purpose of measuring blood pressure of a patient is to evaluate his individual risk of suffering a major cardiovascular complication such as heart attack, stroke, congestive heart failure and renal failure.

Several studies have suggested that ambulatory blood pressure monitoring provides a more accurate evaluation of the risk to an individual patient than the blood pressure measured in the physician's office. Many investigators have found that by using ambulatory blood pressure recordings, the antihypertensive efficacy of a given pharmacologic agent can be evaluated with greater precision than can be achieved using office blood pressure measurements. It also appears that the placebo effect on blood pressure becomes almost negligible when using ambulatory blood pressure monitoring. Still more work is needed to validate these findings. So far also unresolved is the question as to whether blood pressure variability is an independent risk factor. Only non-invasive devices which render monitoring of variability possible on a large scale will open the door to future studies in this area.

Already, ambulatory blood pressure monitoring is taking an increasingly important place in the investigation of hypertensive patients. Though many workers are already convinced that it provides a better evaluation of the cardiovascular risk of a given hypertensive patient, it is probably still too early to make any recommendation for its general use. See also *Arterial blood pressure: Arterial hypertension: Sphygmo-manometer*

Amiloride

A potassium-sparing diuretic used in preference to potassium supplements with thiazide or loop diuretics.
It is also used in higher doses for the medical treatment of primary aldosteronism. Its mechanism of action seems to be the same as that for triamterene. Both drugs interfere with ion

Amiloride

transport in the distal segments of the nephron. The mechanism probably involves reduction of the electrical potential across the tubular epithelial membrane which is one of the major driving forces for potassium secretion.

Amiloride-sensitive sodium-hydrogen ion countertransport
see *Sodium-hydrogen ion countertransport*

Aminoglutethimide
Inhibitor of adrenocortical steroid synthesis acting at the stage of conversion of cholesterol to pregnenolone which has been used to treat patients with adrenocortical carcinoma and Cushing's syndrome.

Amitriptyline
A tricyclic antidepressant which blocks re-uptake of noradrenaline into the nerve ending and may cause orthostatic hypotension. See also *Orthostatic hypotension*

Amphetamine
Drug with powerful central nervous system stimulant actions in addition to the peripheral alpha- and beta-adrenergic stimulant actions common to all indirectly acting sympathomimetics.
Cardiovascular effects include increased systolic and diastolic blood pressure. Heart rate is often reflexly slowed, but with high doses cardiac arrhythmias may occur. Cardiac output is not enhanced by therapeutic doses. Amphetamine and similar drugs were once widely used in the treatment of obesity.

Analgesic nephropathy
Commonest form of chronic drug-induced renal damage.
Chronic ingestion of phenacetin analgesic mixtures causes necrosis of the renal papillae and interstitial nephritis. Papillary necrosis follows the consumption of 1-2 kg of such analgesics. Experimentally large doses of aspirin can give rise to papillary necrosis although the clinical outcome of this is uncertain.
Papillary necrosis has also been described in patients treated with non-steroidal anti-inflammatory drugs. Analgesic nephropathy is more common in females. Clinical features include psychiatric disturbance, anaemia, dyspepsia, ischaemic heart disease, premature ageing, recurrent urinary infections, chronic renal failure and hypertension (50%). Treated by discontinuation of excessive analgesic consumption, but may progress to end-stage renal failure.

Anazolene sodium
Compound used in the measurement of blood volume and cardiac output.

Androstenedione
Androgenic steroid, less potent than testosterone, secreted by testis, adrenal cortex and ovary.

Aneurysm
Swelling produced by dilatation of the wall of an artery, vein, or the heart. Arterial aneurysms are more likely to rupture in the presence of hypertension.
Most fusiform or saccular aneurysms of the thoracic or abdominal aorta are caused by atherosclerosis (Figure 11), but other causes include syphilis, medial necrosis, infective endocarditis and trauma. Dissecting aneurysms result from an intimal tear or intramural haemorrhage in the arterial wall which ruptures into the lumen. Rupture of intracranial arterial aneurysms (berry aneurysms) causes subarachnoid haemorrhage. Cardiac ventricular aneurysms may develop within days of a major myocardial infarction. They may be associated with congestive cardiac failure, ventricular arrhythmias and systemic embolization. See also *Bouchard-Charcot microaneurysms: Dissecting aortic aneurysm*

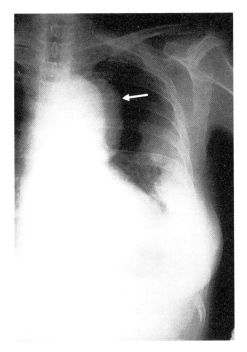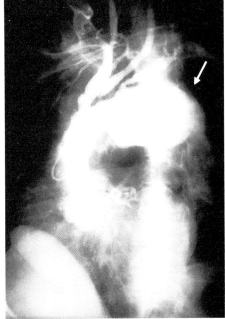

Figure 11(a) **Aneurysm**. Aortic arch aneurysm in a hypertensive patient : chest radiograph showing double aortic shadow (arrowed). Opacification at the left lung base was caused by blood leaking into the pleural space

Figure 11(b) **Aneurysm**. Same patient's arch aortogram showing the lumen of the aneurysm (arrowed). All the major vessels are diffusely atheromatous

ANF
see *Antinuclear factor*

Angiitis
Inflammation of a blood vessel.

Angina pectoris
Chest pain usually provoked by exertion and often associated with coronary artery atherosclerosis. More common in hypertensive patients. Both angina and hypertension may be treated with beta-adrenergic antagonists and calcium antagonists. See also *Atherosclerosis: Ischaemic heart disease: Myocardial infarction*

Angiocardiography (cardioangiography)
Radiological technique in which the heart, great vessels and coronary arteries are demonstrated by the introduction of contrast medium into the circulation. It is most commonly used to demonstrate regions of narrowing of the coronary arteries caused by atherosclerosis.

Angiography (arteriography)
Visualization of blood vessels by injecting contrast medium into them.

Angiometer
Instrument used to measure the diameter of, and tension in, blood vessels.

17

Angio-oedema

Angio-oedema (angioneuroedema, angioedema, angioneurotic oedema)
Condition characterized by recurrent attacks of transient oedema suddenly appearing in areas of the skin, mucous membranes and occasionally viscera. It is related to urticaria and there are various types: idiopathic, IgE-dependent, complement-mediated, those due to agents acting directly on mast cells, those caused by agents altering arachidonic acid metabolism.
Hereditary angio-oedema is of the complement-mediated type and is often associated with abdominal pain. The idiopathic form is by far the commonest class of angio-oedema and is treated with H_1-type antihistamine preparations. Angio-oedema may be a side-effect of some antihypertensive agents, for example, angiotensin I converting enzyme inhibitors.

Angioplasty (arterioplasty)
Repair or reconstruction of a blood vessel. Percutaneous transluminal angioplasty is dilatation of a stenosed vessel, for example, a renal or coronary artery, using a deflated balloon catheter inserted into it followed by inflation of the balloon (Figure 12). See also *Renovascular hypertension*

Angiotensin(s)
A group of peptides present in the blood and elsewhere that have (with the possible exception of angiotensin I) vasoconstrictor properties, and stimulate secretion of aldosterone from the adrenal cortex. See also *Renin-angiotensin system*

Angiotensin I
Decapeptide produced when renin catalyzes the hydrolytic cleavage of angiotensinogen (renin substrate), an alpha-globulin. (Figure 13)

Angiotensin I converting enzyme
(*also known as* ACE: Dipeptidyl carboxypeptidase: Kininase II) A rather nonspecific glycoprotein metalloenzyme (containing one zinc ion per molecule) that

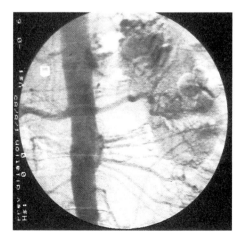

Figure 12(a) Angioplasty. Digital subtraction renal arteriogram showing a tight left renal artery stenosis

Figure 12(b) Angioplasty. Same patient's arteriogram one month after percutaneous angioplasty . The stenosis is no longer present and blood pressure was normal

18

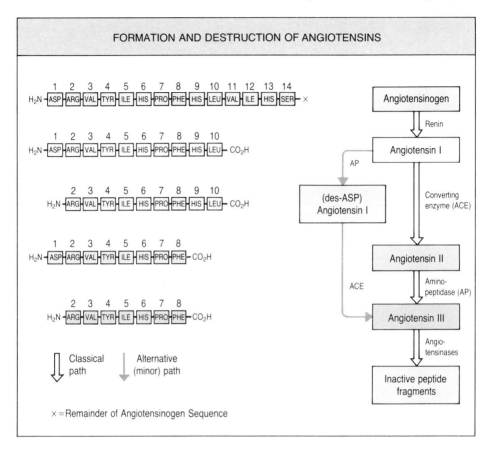

Figure 13 Angiotensin I. Formation and destruction of angiotensins

catalyzes the cleavage of carboxy terminal dipeptide units from peptides with diverse amino acid sequences including angiotensin I. Preferred substrates have one free carboxyl group (but not two) in the C-terminal residue, and proline must not be the penultimate amino acid. This latter feature explains why angiotensin II cannot serve as a substrate. Peptides with proline in the penultimate position act as converting enzyme inhibitors. The enzyme can also be inhibited by chelating agents such as ethylene-diamine-tetra-acetic acid (EDTA), which may act by binding divalent cations such as Ca^{2+} or Zn^{2+} necessary for function.

Orally active converting enzyme inhibitors are thought to bind to the active site in a manner analogous to endogenous substrates. Among the many natural substrates for converting enzyme is bradykinin. Converting enzyme is identical to kininase II which inactivates bradykinin and other potent vasodilator peptides. Converting enzyme appears to be associated with the luminal aspect of vascular endothelial cells in the lungs and other organs, and only a small amount is free in plasma. In Man the lung converts 20-40% of angiotensin I to angiotensin II in a single pass.

Angiotensin I converting enzyme inhibitors

(*also known as* ACE inhibitors)
Angiotensin I converting enzyme (ACE) can be inhibited by certain chelating agents and also by compounds that react with specific side chains of the protein.

Other inhibiting agents
Endogenous peptides that have an inhibitory effect on ACE include beta-lipotrophin. Peptides extracted from the venom of certain snakes (including *Bothrops jararaca*, the Brazilian arrowhead viper) were found to potentiate bradykinin, and subsequently were shown to inhibit ACE. One of these peptides, teprotide, is particularly potent, but none of these agents can be given orally because of inactivation by gastro-intestinal enzymes. The first orally active ACE inhibitor was captopril. This drug and other oral ACE inhibitors are thought to act by binding to the active site in a manner analogous to endogenous substrates. Some side-effects of captopril, particularly taste loss and skin rashes, are similar to side-effects of penicillamine and were attributed to the presence of a sulphydryl group. This led to the development of compounds such as enalapril which does not have a sulphydryl group. Other ACE inhibitors which are soon to be available include solapril, lysinopril and ramipril.

Clinical uses
Orally active ACE inhibitors are effective in lowering blood pressure in patients with renovascular hypertension, although concern has been expressed about the effects of lowering angiotensin II on the function of the kidney with a stenosed artery.
There is good evidence that intrarenal angiotensin II in the affected kidney is responsible for compensatory effects which help sustain glomerular filtration, and, to some extent, the main renal artery pressure distal to the stenosis. These drugs should certainly be avoided in patients with bilateral renovascular disease, as deterioration in overall renal function may result. ACE inhibitors are as effective as beta-blockers or thiazide diuretics in treating essential hypertension. Addition of a diuretic may control the blood pressure of a patient in whom good control was not achieved with an ACE inhibitor alone.

Angiotensin I converting enzyme inhibitors are also effective agents for the treatment of cardiac failure. One feature of this group of drugs is the occasional occurrence of a steep fall in blood pressure following administration of the first dose of the agent. This is particularly likely to occur in patients with high plasma renin activity, for example, those who are sodium depleted or taking drug regimes including diuretics. Treatment should be started with a low dose of the ACE inhibitor, ideally at an interval after withdrawal of the diuretic.

Other mechanisms
As angiotensin I converting enzyme catalyzes reactions other than the formation of angiotensin II, it has been suggested that the antihypertensive effects of ACE inhibitors are not related solely to the lowering of the concentration of angiotensin II. While effects such as potentiation of kinins and stimulation of vasodilator prostaglandins may have some part to play, it seems likely that most of the hypotensive effects are due to inhibition of the conversion of angiotensin I to angiotensin II.

Angiotensin II

An octapeptide formed by the action of angiotensin converting enzyme on angiotensin I, which has numerous effects including the following:

Cardiovascular system Angiotensin II causes vasoconstriction of pre-capillary arterioles and post-capillary venules partly by a direct action and partly via sympathetic stimulation. The vaso-constrictor effect is most potent in the skin, the splanchnic circulation, and the kidney. Angiotensin II also has a positive

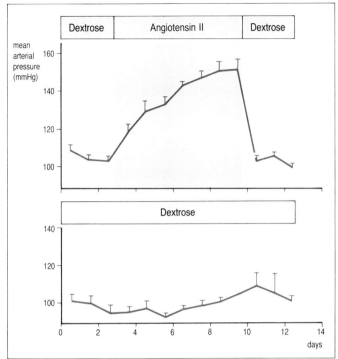

Figure 14 Angiotensin II.
Angiotensin II has a slow pressor effect: (upper) Effect on mean arterial pressure of conscious unrestrained rats of infusion of angiotensin II at a constant and initially sub-pressor rate, that is, at a rate which did not increase blood pressure acutely: (lower) Control infusion of dextrose in similar rats. Mean arterial pressure in the rats infused with angiotensin II rises by 50 mmHg over seven days

inotropic effect on the heart, but no direct effect on heart rate. Angiotensin II has a potent acute pressor action, and there is also a slow pressor effect evident with prolonged infusion (Figure 14).

Central nervous system Angiotensin II cannot cross the blood brain barrier but in the systemic circulation it can act on the circumventricular organs. Angiotensin II infused into the vertebral arteries can cause central sympathetic stimulation with vasoconstriction and cardiac stimulation resulting from its effects on the area postrema. Dipsogenic effects can be caused by intravenous or intracerebroventricular injection. Injection into the third ventricle or supraphysiological concentrations of angiotensin II in the peripheral circulation can stimulate release of antidiuretic hormone from the posterior pituitary.

Peripheral autonomic nervous system

Angiotensin II can facilitate peripheral sympathetic transmission mainly by increasing the output of noradrenaline from nerve terminals.

Adrenal medulla Angiotensin II stimulates the release of catecholamines by causing depolarization of the chromaffin cells.

Adrenal cortex Angiotensin II stimulates the synthesis and secretion of aldosterone. Its effect on the production of other corticosteroids is variable and usually minor.

Kidney Angiotensin II has direct actions on the kidney, in addition to the effects on sodium and potassium handling mediated by aldosterone. The general pressor effect plus constriction of the efferent arteriole will tend to increase glomerular filtration. Constriction of the afferent arteriole will tend to have the opposite effect. The net result depends to some degree on the

21

Angiotensin II

concentration of angiotensin II.

Effects on prostaglandin metabolism
Angiotensin II and bradykinin can stimulate phospholipase A_2 causing release of arachidonic acid from membrane phospholipids. This is the initial step in the synthesis of a variety of prostaglandins some of which have vasoconstrictor and others vasodilator effects.

Angiotensin II antagonists

Peptides which compete with angiotensin II for its receptor, but do not (in the case of pure antagonists), on binding to the receptor, produce the physiological response.

Agonist activity is greatly reduced by replacement of phenylalanine at the 8 position. Saralasin has this feature, and the substitution of sarcosine at position 1 slows degradation of the peptide and increases its affinity for the receptor. Saralasin is actually a partial agonist, and commonly causes a transient rise in blood pressure when given intravenously to normal subjects or patients with hypertension. The subsequent effect on blood pressure depends largely on the prevailing concentration of angiotensin II (in general, saralasin lowers blood pressure if angiotensin II concentration is raised). Some patients in whom blood pressure falls acutely at this stage have marked rebound hypertension 1-3 hours later. This unpredictability has limited the therapeutic usefulness of angiotensin II antagonists, but their specificity has made them useful for studying the renin-angiotensin system.

Angiotensin II pressor system

A system in the rat forebrain which mediates the central pressor response to angiotensin II and is involved in the development of renin-dependent hypertension. See also *Anteroventral third ventricle: Brain renin-angiotensin system*

Angiotensin II-reducing drugs

Plasma concentration of angiotensin II may be lowered by drugs acting at a number of sites.

Beta-adrenergic antagonists, among their many actions, suppress secretion of renin and thereby reduce angiotensin I and II. Renin inhibitors decrease the enzymatic conversion of angiotensinogen to angiotensin I.

Inhibitors of angiotensin I converting enzyme also lower angiotensin II, but in this case angiotensin I concentration is increased.

Angiotensin III

Heptapeptide formed when an aminopeptidase catalyzes the hydrolysis of angiotensin II. It shares most of the properties of angiotensin II, but is generally less potent with the possible exception of the effects on the adrenal cortex.

Angiotensin receptors

(special contribution from Dr J. McQueen, Medical Research Council Blood Pressure Unit, Glasgow, Scotland).

Receptors for angiotensin II are localized to the plasma membrane of the following cell types which are specified in Table 3. In all tissues the receptor exhibits the same selectivity for angiotensin peptides (potency series; angiotensin II > angiotensin III >> angiotensin I) and may be blocked by competitive inhibitors (for example, saralasin and sar[1] thr[8] angiotensin II).

The C-terminal pentapeptide of angiotensin II is essential for binding to the receptor to occur. In several tissues the receptor has been characterized as a sulphydryl-sensitive dimeric glycoprotein (subunit M_r 68000).

Angiotensin action is associated with increased transmembrane sodium flux and mobilization of intracellular calcium and is dependent on calcium influx. The angiotensin receptor appears to be coupled via a guanosine triphosphate-binding protein to phospholipase C, stimulating hydrolysis of phosphatidylinositol bisphosphate to inositol trisphosphate (releases calcium from endoplasmic reticulum) and diacylglycerol (acts through protein kinase C to activate an amiloride-sensitive sodium/proton exchange channel).

Alteration of plasma angiotensin II concentration causes a reciprocal change in the number of angiotensin receptors per cell in most tissues, with corresponding changes in target organ sensitivity to the peptide. Desensitization in resistance vessels is particularly marked. In contrast steroidogenic responsiveness and the number of receptors per zona glomerulosa cell vary directionally with the plasma angiotensin II concentration. Other hormones (oestrogen, progesterone, aldosterone, insulin) may affect angiotensin receptor numbers in certain tissues. See also *Angiotensin II: Angiotensin II antagonists: Inositol lipid metabolism*

Angiotensinases
A group of peptides in plasma which catalyze the hydrolysis of angiotensins to inactive peptide fragments. (Figure 13)

Angiotensinogen
(*also known as* Renin substrate) A glycoprotein synthesized in the liver and present in abundance in the alpha-globulin fraction of the plasma proteins. Angiotensinogen acts as a substrate for renin, which catalyzes the cleavage of angiotensin I from the amino terminus of angiotensinogen. The human protein serves as a substrate only for the renin of man or primates, whereas angiotensinogens of other animals serve as substrates for the renins of many species, including man. Glucocorticoids increase the rate of synthesis of the protein, and increased plasma concentrations are found in Cushing's syndrome, and in patients receiving ACTH or corticosteroids. Angiotensinogen synthesis is also increased by oestrogens, and greatly elevated plasma concentrations may be found in pregnant women, and in those taking the combined oral contraceptive pill. Low plasma levels of angiotensinogen may be found in patients with Addison's disease, or in those who have had an adrenalectomy.

Angiotonia
Vascular tone.

Angiotonic
Increasing vascular tone.

Antagonist
Agent which binds to a receptor, but does not cause a physiological response. Interferes with the effect of an agonist.

Table 3 Angiotensin receptors

Tissue	Cell / organ response to receptors
Vascular smooth muscle	Vasoconstriction, especially in resistance vessels of cutaneous, splanchnic and renal vasculature
Zona glomerulosa of the adrenal cortex	Aldosterone secretion
Adrenal medulla	Catecholamine release
Myocardium	Positive inotropic effect
Renal glomeruli and tubules	Haemodynamic effects, altered tubular sodium transport; inhibition of renin release
Circumventricular organs of brain	Dipsogenic and cardiovascular effects Vasopressin release; Increased sympathetic discharge
Liver	Glycogenolysis
Platelets	Increased sensitivity to aggregation

Anteroventral third ventricle (AV3V)

Anteroventral third ventricle (AV3V)

Region in the hypothalamus of the rat which is part of the angiotensin II pressor system of the rat forebrain. Intracerebroventricular administration of angiotensin II normally has a pressor effect and lesions of the AV3V region abolish this.

Antidiuretic hormone

(*also known as* ADH) (special contribution from Dr P. L. Padfield, Western General Hospital, Edinburgh, Scotland)

Arginine vasopressin

Arginine vasopressin is the human form of the antidiuretic hormone. Secreted by the paraventricular and supraoptic nuclei of the hypothalamus it is stored in the neurohypothesis (posterior pituitary gland) and under normal circumstances is released following an increase in plasma osmolality. A 1% change in plasma osmolality is sufficient to alter ADH release, there being a relatively linear relationship with plasma osmolality between osmolality levels of 280 and 295 mOsm/kg. Normal circulating levels of vasopressin in man range from 0.5 to 5 pg/ml (0.5-5 pmol/l). Vasopressin renders the cells of the distal nephron and collecting duct permeable to water thus allowing osmotic reabsorption and the production of a concentrated urine. It is by this means that water is conserved. If further dehydration occurs above plasma osmolalities of 295 then thirst is activated to increase water intake. A deficiency of ADH leads to thirst and polyuria (cranial diabetes insipidus). Excess secretion results in excessive water retention with hyponatraemia, the syndrome of inappropriate antidiuretic hormone release.

Vasopressin

As its name implies vasopressin is also a potent constrictor of vascular smooth muscle; more powerful even than angiotensin II. Despite this, infused vasopressin is only capable of raising blood pressure in normal subjects when plasma levels of approximately 100 pg/ml are reached. Lower levels do induce vasoconstriction, however, particularly in the skin and splanchnic vessels such that total peripheral resistance is increased. Blood pressure is prevented from rising by a concomitant fall in cardiac output brought about by a marked decrease in heart rate. The importance of the autonomic nervous system for this buffering action is strikingly demonstrated in patients with autonomic nervous failure where the pressor response to infused vasopressin is enhanced between 100 and 1000 fold.

Vasopressin is released following volume depletion or acute blood loss irrespective of plasma osmolality levels and may circulate in amounts greater than 100 pg/ml. At this level vasopressin is important in raising blood pressure in conjunction with angiotensin II. Its selective effects preserve renal blood flow in contradistinction to the effects of angiotensin II.

Several animal models of hypertension have been associated with raised circulating levels of vasopressin and the administration of vasopressin antibodies or antagonists has often resulted in dramatic falls in blood pressure. Circulating levels of vasopressin are not however elevated in patients with benign essential hypertension. Indeed, the release of vasopressin for a given increase in plasma osmolality is less marked in the presence of hypertension than in normal subjects (the opposite of that seen in hypotensive or hypovolaemic states). There is no evidence for an increased sensitivity to the pressor effects of vasopressin in hypertensive subjects. In some forms of severe hypertension, particularly in the malignant phase, vasopressin levels are elevated but this is likely to be a consequence of the disorder rather than the cause. See also *Collecting ducts: Diabetes insipidus: Nephron: Syndrome of inappropriate ADH secretion*

Table 4 Classification of antihypertensive drugs

Site of action	Drug
Central sites	Reserpine Rauwolfia Derivatives Alpha-methyldopa Clonidine
Ganglion blockers	Mecamylamine Pempidine Hexamethonium Pentolinium
Adrenergic neurone blockers	Debrisoquine Bethanidine Guanethidine
Beta adrenergic blockers: Selective	Atenolol Metoprolol Acebutolol
Non-selective	Oxprenolol Pindolol Timolol Propranolol etc.
Alpha adrenergic blockers	Prazosin Phentolamine Phenoxybenzamine
Alpha and beta adrenergic blockers	Labetalol
Vasodilators	Hydralazine Minoxidil Nitroprusside Diazoxide
Diuretics: Thiazides	Bendrofluazide Cyclopenthiazide Chlorthalidone etc.
Loop	Frusemide Bumetanide Ethacrynic acid
Potassium-sparing	Spironolactone Amiloride Triamterene
Calcium antagonists	Nifedipine Verapamil etc.
Angiotensin I converting enzyme inhibitors	Captopril Enalapril

Antihypertensive drugs
Drugs which lower blood pressure by various mechanisms (Table 4). See also *Adrenergic neurone blocking agents: Alpha-adrenergic receptor blocking drugs: Angiotensin I converting enzyme inhibitors: Beta-adrenergic receptor blocking drugs: Calcium antagonists: Centrally acting antihypertensive drugs: Diuretics: Ganglion blocking drugs: Renin inhibitors: Vasodilators*

Antihypertensive drugs and serum lipids
Certain drugs used to treat hypertension can alter serum lipid and lipoprotein levels (Table 5).
Thiazide diuretics tend to increase total serum cholesterol, low density lipoprotein cholesterol and total serum triglyceride concentrations. Studies have shown increased total serum triglyceride concentration and decreased high density lipoprotein cholesterol in patients taking beta-adrenergic receptor blocking drugs. The alpha-adrenergic antagonist prazosin lowers total serum cholesterol concentration and may increase high density lipoprotein cholesterol level (both potentially beneficial effects). It has not, however, been formally proven that any of the potentially adverse or beneficial effects of antihypertensive drugs on serum lipids affect cardiovascular risk.

Antihypertensive neutral renomedullary lipid (ANRL)
This is the main putative hormone of the renomedullary interstitial cells. It is a lipid secreted by the renomedullary interstitial cells that appears relatively non-polar on chromatography.
ANRL acts as a vasodilator that causes bradycardia and decreased sympathetic output and these effects are produced by renal venous effluent after unclipping in the one clip, one kidney hypertensive rat.

Antihypertensive polar renomedullary lipid (APRL)
A mixture of alkyl ether analogues of phosphatidylcholine with an acetoyl group

Antihypertensive polar renomedullary lipid (APRL)

Table 5 Antihypertensive drugs and serum lipids

	Total Cholesterol (per cent)	High Density Lipoprotein Cholesterol (per cent)	Low Density Lipoprotein Cholesterol (per cent)	Triglycerides (per cent)
Thiazide diuretics	↑5 - 8	—	↑5 - 8	↑15 - 25
Beta blockers	—	↓10	—	↑30
Alpha blockers	↓5 - 8	—	—	—

at position 2 on Figure 15 secreted by the renomedullary interstitial cells. APRL acts as a vasodilator, but (unlike ANRL) causes tachycardia and increased sympathetic nervous system activity in the rat. See also *Antihypertensive neutral renomedullary lipid: Antihypertensive renomedullary lipids*

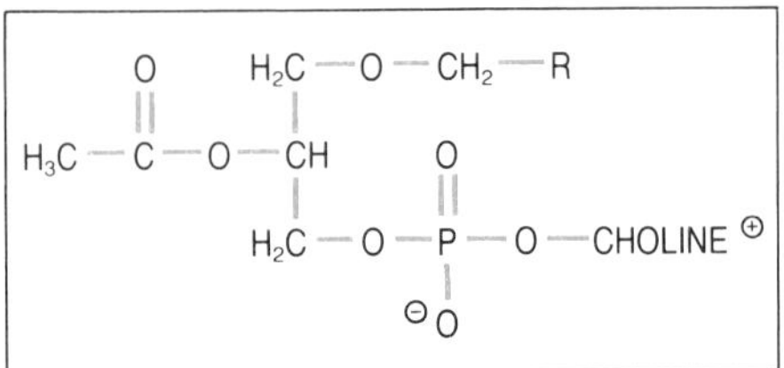

Antihypertensive Polar Renomedullary Lipid (R=Alkyl group)

Figure 15 APRL. General structure of anti-hypertensive polar renomedullary lipid (R = alkyl group)

Antihypertensive renomedullary lipids

Cells of the renal papilla (inner medulla), known as the renomedullary interstitial cells (RIC) secrete a substance (or substances) with an antihypertensive action.

Two classes of antihypertensive lipids are secreted by RIC in culture and can be detected in renal venous effluent after unclipping in the one kidney, one clip hypertensive rat. These are the anti-hypertensive polar and the anti-

hypertensive neutral renomedullary lipids. Many of the effects of the reno-medullary substance are antagonistic to those of angiotensin II. See also *Renal disease causing hypertension*

Antinatriuresis

Prevention of sodium excretion in the urine.

Antinuclear factor (ANF)

ANF refers to a group of antibodies directed against any of the antigenic constituents of the nucleus: for instance, antibodies to double stranded DNA are found in high titre in systemic lupus erythematosus and in low titre in other rheumatic diseases. In drug-induced lupus the screening test for ANF is positive but anti-double stranded DNA is negative. See also *Drug-induced lupus*

Antirheumatic drugs

Drugs used in rheumatic disease, for example, indomethacin which antagonizes the antihypertensive effect of propranolol and thiazides, possibly by interference with renal prostaglandin metabolism. See also *Indomethacin*

Aorta

The principal trunk from which the systemic arterial system branches. The ascending aorta arises from the left ventricle of the heart and joins the aortic arch. The descending aorta arises from the aortic arch in the thorax and passes through the diaphragm into the abdomen. The descending aorta bifurcates at about the level of the fourth lumbar vertebra to form the common iliac arteries.

Aortic baroreceptor
see *Arterial baroreceptors*

Aortic baroreceptor deafferentation (ABD)
Removal of the afferent nerve supply to the aortic baroreceptor in a conscious rat produces hypertension acutely. Ganglion blockade in these animals causes an exaggerated fall in blood pressure, which suggests that the hypertension was due to increased sympathetic activity. This enhanced activity is less evident several weeks after ABD when blood pressure returns towards the control level.

Aortic compliance
see *Arterial compliance*

Aortic distensibility
Synonymous with aortic compliance.

Aortic incompetence
(*also known as* Aortic regurgitation) The back flow of blood from the aorta into the left ventricle in diastole.
A murmur compatible with incompetence of the aortic valve may occur rarely with high blood pressure and resolve when pressure is controlled.

Aortic stenosis
Narrowing of the aortic valve.
The peripheral signs of aortic stenosis may be obscured by the presence of co-existing hypertension, especially in the elderly.

Aprotinin (Trasylol)
Polypeptide protease inhibitor often used to inhibit proteolytic degradation of biologically active peptides in blood samples.

Arachidonic acid
(*also known as* 5,8,11,14-Eicosatetraenoic

acid) Polyunsaturated 20-carbon essential fatty acid which is either ingested in meat or derived from dietary linoleic acid. The major precursor in humans of prostaglandins, prostacyclin, thromboxane A_2 and leukotrienes.

Area postrema
Medullary circumventricular organ implicated as a prominent site of action for angiotensin in the dog, cat and rabbit, but not the rat. When angiotensin II is infused in these three species via the vertebral arteries, pressor responses can be demonstrated that are abolished by lesions of the area postrema. See also *Circumventricular organs*

Argipressin
(*also known as* 8-α-arginine vasopressin) Vasopressin with arginine at the 8-position as in the human form. See also *Antidiuretic hormone: Desmopressin: Lypressin*

Arterenol
Synonym for noradrenaline.

Arterial baroreceptors
The arterial baroreceptors are located in the carotid sinus, a dilatation of the internal carotid artery near its origin, and in the wall of the arch of the aorta. Afferent nerve fibres from the carotid sinus travel in the glossopharyngeal nerve, whereas those from the aortic arch travel in the vagus nerve. See also *Baroreceptors and hypertension*

Arterial blood pressure
Pressure of blood within the arteries. In the aorta and large arteries pressure rises to a peak value (systolic pressure) during each cardiac cycle and falls to a minimum value (diastolic pressure). Pulse pressure is the difference between the systolic and diastolic pressures. Mean pressure is the average value throughout the cardiac cycle. It can actually be determined only by integrating the area

Arterial blood pressure

under the pressure curve, but an approximate value is given by adding one third of the pulse pressure to the diastolic pressure.

Arterial compliance
(special contribution from Professor A. Simon and Dr J. Levenson, Centre de Diagnostic de l'Hôpital Broussais, Paris.)
Definition
Compliance is a general term describing change in dimension of an elastic material with a change in stress. When applied to arteries, compliance is the ratio of the change in volume ($\triangle V$) resulting from a change in transmural distending pressure ($\triangle P$) or $\triangle V/\triangle P$, that is, the slope of the pressure-volume relationship. Such a relationship is curvilinear because of the non-linear distensible characteristics of arteries. This means that compliance must decrease with increasing

pressure, so that the transmural pressure at which compliance is measured must be specified. Moreover, compliance should be estimated on small pressure changes. Although arterial compliance is determined by elastic vessel properties, it is not itself a true measure of elasticity which refers to an elastic modulus (stress-strain ratio) usually measured circumferentially for a hollow cylindrical artery. Compliance is, however, invaluable when determining the volumic reservoir role of the aorta and major arteries. Mathematically speaking, compliance ($\triangle V/\triangle P$) equals the product of arterial volume (V) and the relative volumic distensibility ($\triangle V/V\triangle P$). The latter depends on the intrinsic elastic properties of the arterial walls, as demonstrated by the classical equation of pulse wave velocity (C) C = $(V\triangle P/\rho\triangle V)^{1/2}$, ($\rho$ being the blood density), described by Thomas

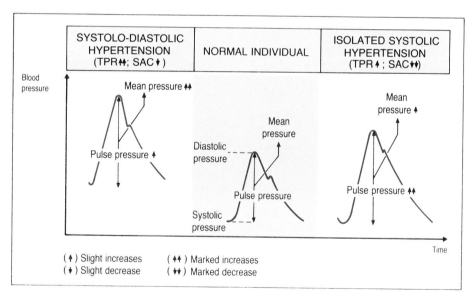

Figure 16 Arterial compliance. Intra-arterial pressure recorded as a function of time (as might be obtained via a catheter in the brachial artery) in (a) a patient with raised systolic and diastolic blood pressure; (b) a normal individual; and (c) a patient with isolated systolic hypertension. The changes in total peripheral resistance (TPR) and systemic arterial compliance (SAC) are indicated

Young from Isaac Newton's experiments that related velocity of sound in air to its bulk elastic modulus.

Therefore, arterial compliance takes into account vessel geometry and the intrinsic elastic properties of the arteries. By regulating the sequestration of blood in the large distended arteries during systole, arterial compliance damps down the pulsatility of pressure and flow generated by the heart. This is analogous to the simple Windkessel model of the circulation which compared the arterial system to the air chamber of early fire engines.

As peripheral resistance determines mean arterial pressure in relation to mean cardiac output, so arterial compliance is responsible for the amplitude of the pulse pressure in relation to intermittent cardiac ejection (Figure 16). Thus, for a given pulsatile pump, the lower the arterial compliance, the higher the pulsatility of systemic pressure.

Results in hypertension
In human studies, advances in Doppler measurements of flow and the diameter of arteries have led to two experimental approaches. Firstly, the analysis of pressure and flow using a Windkessel model of the circulation permits calculation of compliance from the exponential diastolic pressure decay slope. Secondly, the determination of pulse wave velocity (C) and luminal radius (R) of one arterial segment allows calculation of compliance per unit length of one artery as the $(\pi R^2/\rho C^2)$ ratio, ρ being the density of blood.

These methods have shown that reduction in arterial compliance is the hall-mark of the effect of hypertension on large arteries, but this phenomenon is not exclusively due to blood pressure elevation which stiffens arterial walls by increasing their stretch. Arterial compliance is decreased early in borderline to mild hypertension, suggesting the participation of functional and/or structural changes in arteries, independent of the effect of raised blood pressure *per se*. Reduction in compliance impairs the buffering function of the circulation and increases the pulsatility of pressure. This is apparent in systolic hypertension in the elderly where arterial compliance is negatively correlated with pulse and systolic pressures.

Hyperpulsatile pressure waves may chronically fatigue arterial bioelastomers and increase cardiac work, so that the response of arterial compliance to antihypertensive treatment should be taken into account in the therapeutic approach to hypertension.

See also *Haemodynamics of systemic hypertension*

Arterial endothelium
Layer of epithelial cells that lines the arteries. It is capable of numerous essential biological functions. Removal of endothelium *in vitro* often leads to altered vasoconstrictor response of vessel to a number of agents.

Arterial hypertension
Raised blood pressure within the (systemic) arterial tree.

Hypertension may be defined as a blood pressure more than an arbitrary number of standard deviations (say two) above the mean value for age and sex. However, the term is probably better defined in terms of risk: for example, the level of blood pressure above which treatment can be shown to be beneficial (reducing the risk of disease without causing unacceptable side-effects). Prognosis is as much linked to systolic as to diastolic pressure, and the mean pressure may be the value which best predicts the degree of end-organ damage. One classification of hypertension which has been proposed is set out in Table 6. Most large studies suggest that three or more readings by the same observer in similar surroundings over a four-month period are required to establish the level of an individual's blood pressure. Hypertensives are at increased

Arterial hypertension

risk of cerebrovascular disease, ischaemic heart disease, cardiac failure and renal failure. See also *Arterial blood pressure: Complications of hypertension*

Table 6 Classification of arterial hypertension

1. Normotension

(a) Age 17 - 40 years:
blood pressure
< 140 / 90 mm Hg.

(b) Age 41 - 60 years:
blood pressure
< 150 / 90 mm Hg.

(c) Age over 60 years:
blood pressure
< 160 / 90 mm Hg.

2.Hypertension

(a) Age 17 - 60 years:
blood pressure
> 160 / 100 mm Hg.

(b) Age over 60 years:
blood pressure
> 175 / 100 mm Hg.

3.Borderline hypertension

Readings between the hypertensive and normotensive values

Arterial hypertension as a cause of renal impairment
see *Renal disease causing hypertension*

Arterial smooth muscle
see *Vascular smooth muscle*

Arterial wall
The wall of an artery consists of three layers:

Tunica intima is the internal layer lined by squamous endothelial cells. Sub-endothelial elements are orientated longitudinally. The *tunica intima* is separated from the *tunica media* by the fenestrated internal elastic lamina.

Tunica media is the thickest layer containing varying proportions of muscular and elastic elements arranged in a direction circular to the vessel. The *tunica media* is separated from the *tunica adventitia* by the external elastic lamina.

Tunica adventitia gradually merges with loose connective tissue.

Arteriography
see *Angiography*

Arteriole
A minute arterial branch. The wall of an arteriole contains proportionally much more smooth muscle than that of an artery. The term is particularly applied to the vessel just proximal to the capillary. The muscle is innervated by adrenergic nerve fibres and in some cases cholinergic fibres. The arterioles are the main site of resistance to blood flow and small changes in their calibre cause large changes in total peripheral resistance.

Arterioplasty
see *Angioplasty*

Arteriosclerosis
Diffuse change in the wall of arteries in which the muscle and elastic tissue diminishes and is replaced by fibrous tissue with the result that the arteries become more rigid. Occurs to various degrees with ageing, but is accelerated by systemic arterial hypertension and cigarette smoking. See also *Athero-sclerosis*

Arteriosclerosis obliterans
(*also known as* Endarteritis obliterans, if it is found in chronic inflammatory lesions) Arteriosclerosis in which proliferation of the *tunica intima* of small arteries has

caused complete obliteration of the lumen.

Arteriosclerotic retinopathy
see *Hypertensive retinopathy*

Arteriosympathectomy
Removal of the sheath of an artery containing the sympathetic fibres to produce temporary vasodilatation.

Arteriovenous nipping
A feature of hypertensive retinopathy in which the hypertrophied arteries partially interrupt the column of blood in the veins due to compression of the latter within the common adventitia (Figure 17).

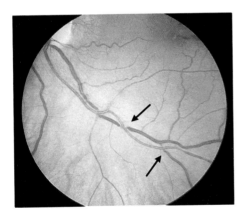

Figure 17 Arteriovenous nipping (arrowed)

Arteritis
Inflammation of an artery.

Artery
Vessel through which blood flows on its way from the heart to the periphery. Large arteries are elastic, whereas medium-sized and small arteries are muscular.

Ask-Upmark kidney
(Erik Ask-Upmark 1901-1968)
(*also known as* Segmental renal hypoplasia) Unilateral segmental renal hypoplasia is a rare condition which is commoner in females. It is a cause of hypertension in children and is frequently associated with vesicoureteric reflux. The small kidney has one or more scarred lobes and renal venous measurements of renin show increased secretion on the affected side. Removal of the abnormal kidney usually cures the hypertension.

Aspartyl proteases
A group of enzymes which includes renin, cathepsin D and pepsin, which catalyze hydrolysis of protein substrates and have two aspartyl residues involved in the catalytic site.
There are strong similarities between the amino acid sequences and x-ray studies have shown that these proteins have a bilobar structure with a well-defined cleft. The two aspartyl residues lie close together on either side of the cleft. Renin differs from the other aspartyl proteases in its higher catalytic optimum pH and its extreme substrate specificity.

Aspirin
(*also known as* Acetylsalicylic acid)
Anti-inflammatory agent and analgesic used in low dose (150-300 mg daily) for prevention of transient ischaemic attacks. In the latter situation the drug is acting as an inhibitor of platelet aggregation. It achieves this by acetylating enzymes involved in the synthesis of prostaglandins.

Asthma
Variable narrowing of the airways which can be precipitated or made worse by administration of beta-adrenergic antagonists, especially of the non-selective type.

Atenolol
Long-acting cardioselective beta-adrenergic antagonist. See also *Beta-adrenergic receptor blocking drugs*

Atherogenesis
Formation of atheromatous plaques.

Atherosclerosis

(special contribution from Professor
M.J. Davies, British Heart Foundation,
Cardiovascular Pathology Unit, London,
England)

Definition

An intimal disease of medium and large
arteries in which there is proliferation of
smooth muscle cells and connective tissue
associated with the deposition of lipid
derived from the plasma.

The intimal proliferation is focal leading
to the formation of atheromatous
plaques. The smallest lesions (fatty
streaks) are focal collections of lipid
filled macrophages within the intima but
larger lesions are oval dome-shaped humps
(raised plaques) in which there is
abundant connective tissue. Raised
plaques may contain small amounts of
lipid only within macrophages (hard
plaques) or contain a large mass of
extracellular lipid (soft plaques). These
lipid-rich soft plaques contain a pool of free
cholesterol and esters encapsulated within
the intima and separated from the arterial
lumen by a cap of fibrous tissue over
which there is intact endothelial surface.

Clinical symptoms

These arise both because the connective
tissue proliferation inherent to atheroma
slowly encroaches on the lumen of the
artery, and because sudden episodes of
thrombosis develop on the plaque
becoming the final common pathway to
a number of acute clinical syndromes.

Thrombosis may be mural, that is,
projecting into the vascular lumen but
not totally preventing flow, or occlusive.
The former type of thrombus may be
responsible for distal platelet microemboli
known to cause transient cerebral
ischaemic attacks and unstable angina.
Occlusive thrombosis is responsible for
such conditions as acute myocardial or
cerebral infarction.

Thrombosis is most frequently invoked
by the process of fissuring, cracking or
rupture of a plaque containing a pool of
extracellular lipid. The fibrous cap of such

a plaque breaks open to allow blood to
enter the lipid pool within the intima. A
mass of thrombus forms as the result of
an interaction between platelets and both
exposed collagen fibrils and free lipid. This
thrombus is initially contained within the
intima and the plaque expands in size. The
plaque may reseal at this stage leaving an
increased degree of residual stenosis. In
other instances additional thrombosis
begins to develop within the lumen over
the fissure and finally may totally occlude
the vessel. Such intraluminal thrombi
involve both fibrin and platelets. Total
thrombotic occlusion is more common in
arteries of the calibre of the coronary and
cerebral while mural thrombus is more
common in the carotid arteries and aorta.

Relation to hypertension

Epidemiologic studies show clearly that
elevated blood pressure is associated with
an increased risk of death from coronary
and cerebral artery disease.

In the *International Atherosclerosis
Project* (IAP) comparison was made
between the amount of atheroma present
at autopsy in the intima of the coronary
arteries and aorta in different geographic
areas throughout the world. Hypertensives
had consistently more fatty streaks and
raised plaques than non-hypertensive
subjects. This was true both in subjects
dying of atheroma-related disease and
those dying of non-vascular causes.
Studies of single populations such as in
Oslo and Hawaii confirm that the
positive correlation coefficient between
the amount of intima involved by plaques
and the systolic blood pressure is
significant at the 1% level.

Hypertensive subjects may therefore be at
greater risk of the clinical manifestations
of atheroma simply because they possess
more plaques. An additional factor may be
a greater propensity of lipid rich plaques to
undergo fissuring and thus thrombosis in
hypertensive subjects.

It is logical that a process which
involves the rupture of a collagenous
structure would be enhanced by elevated

haemodynamic pressures but no proof exists for this view outside the fact that complicated plaques which have undergone thrombosis are also more common in hypertensive than non-hypertensive subjects in the IAP study. The lack of a clear effect in reducing the incidence of acute coronary events by lowering blood pressure is however somewhat against the view that hypertension invokes plaque fissures.

The incremental effect of hypertension on human atherosclerotic lesions is supported by animal work. In hypertensive animals the atherogenic effect of diet-induced hyperlipidaemia is enhanced when the blood pressure is elevated. The role of hypertension in enhancing atheroma has been linked in both man and animals to the interaction of increased pressure on the vessel wall, in particular the endothelial cells. A direct damaging effect on the endothelial surface by pressure and flow is suggested by the selective nature of atheroma for high pressure areas, that is, proximal but not distal to a coarctation of the aorta. Atheroma is seen in the pulmonary arteries in man only in association with pulmonary hypertension.

High intravascular pressure is associated in animals with increased lipid transport across the intima either due to hydrostatic force or an increase in endothelial permeability. Smooth muscle lysosomal enzymes are increased in hypertension possibly reflecting a greater flux of substances such as lipids across the vessel wall.

Atherosclerosis and aneurysms
In the abdominal aorta, atheroma is associated with aneurysm formation rather than stenosis. While atheroma is primarily an intimal disease the media behind plaques undergoes secondary atrophy and finally vanishes. The cause has been postulated to be a reduction of O_2 diffusion across the thickened intima, mechanical pressure or enzymes such as elastases are then released from lipid-filled macrophages within the intima.

If the atheromatous plaques are almost confluent in the intima the whole media may vanish allowing aneurysms to develop. Hypertension is therefore related to aneurysm formation in the abdominal aorta both by virtue of increasing the number of intimal plaques and expanding the aneurysm sac once the media has been lost.

Atherosclerotic cardiovascular disease

Disease in which atherosclerosis affects the coronary and peripheral circulation. Often present in an accelerated form in hypertensive patients. Atherosclerosis affecting the limb vessels causes intermittent claudication which may progress to pain at rest and a gangrenous limb. See also *Angina pectoris: Atherosclerotic heart disease*

Atherosclerotic heart disease

Disease in which atherosclerosis affects the coronary circulation producing reversible ischaemia and angina pectoris. May progress to myocardial infarction.

Atrial natriuretic peptides (ANP)

(special contribution from Dr A.M. Richards, The Princess Margaret Hospital, Christchurch, New Zealand)

Definition
Atrial natriuretic peptides (ANP) possess natriuretic and vasorelaxant qualities which have stimulated ongoing research in many centres in order to determine their role in the regulation of body fluid volumes and arterial pressure.

The peptides are stored in specific granules found in the sarcoplasmic core of mammalian atrial cardiocytes. DNA cloning techniques have permitted description of the amino acid sequence of the peptide precursor in several species including man. Precursors in man, rat, mouse, dog and rabbit contain very similar sequences of approximately 150 amino acids. It seems likely that the predominant

Atrial natriuretic peptides (ANP)

circulating form is the 28 amino acid carboxy terminal fragment.

Effects

Since 1981 the potent natriuretic and diuretic effects of administered atrial extracts and pure synthetic peptides have been confirmed in several species including man. ANP has also been shown to lower arterial pressure and to inhibit secretion of renin and aldosterone and antidiuretic hormone. However, studies to date have involved pharmacological doses of ANP, and how responses to such doses relate to the true physiological and pathophysiological role of the endogenous circulating peptide remains unclear.

Mechanisms

Increases in atrial pressure constitute an important stimulus for the release of ANP into the circulation. Hence it has been postulated that this hormone system

participates in a biological feedback loop in which increased circulating volume raises intra-atrial pressure causing enhanced release of ANP with consequent reduction in atrial pressure secondary to the peptide's receptor-mediated natriuretic and vasodepressor effects (Figure 18).

Clinical features

In support of this hypothesis, sensitive radioimmunoassays have detected enhanced plasma concentrations of ANP in a number of fluid-loaded states including congestive heart failure and primary aldosteronism (Conn's syndrome).

Further, ANP values shift concordantly with changes in the sodium status of normal subjects whether induced by acute intravenous isotonic fluid challenge or by alterations in dietary sodium intake. Clearly a hormone with effects on

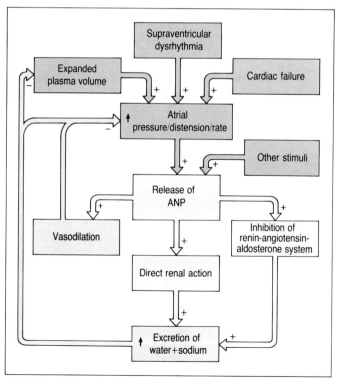

Figure 18
Atrial natriuretic peptides.
Possible roles of atrial natriuretic peptide in body fluid volume and blood pressure homeostasis

vascular tone, renal sodium excretion, and the activity of the renin-angiotensin-aldosterone system, is likely to be involved in the regulation of arterial pressure and may play a role in the pathophysiology of hypertension. Plasma ANP concentrations are elevated in spontaneously hypertensive rats and in a proportion of patients with essential hypertension. Such enhanced levels seem likely to represent a compensatory response, possibly to impaired renal sodium excretory capacity and/or the reduced venous compliance and increased central blood volumes and pressures found in part of the hypertensive population.

Whether varied forms of hypertension are attributable, in part or whole, to deficiencies of ANP synthesis and release or to impaired end organ responses remains to be determined.

ANP or its analogues may provide a new form of pharmacotherapy for hypertension and heart failure. They offer the possibility of inducing diuresis and reducing cardiac pre- and after-loads without inducing a potentially deleterious response from the renin-angiotensin-aldosterone system. Clearly the pitfalls of such therapy, including the risk of severe sodium and fluid depletion, need to be explored in extended trials.

In summary, this newly-discovered cardiac-based hormonal system has a potentially important role in body fluid volume and arterial pressure homeostasis, and may offer in future a therapeutic option in the management of hypertension and heart failure. See also *Aldosteronism: Antidiuretic hormone: Natriuresis: Renin-angiotensin system*

Atropine

An antagonist acting at the muscarinic receptors.

Atropine has numerous effects, including increasing heart rate by blocking the effect of the vagus nerve on the sinoatrial node of the heart. It may be useful in tests

of parasymnpathetic function. See also *Autonomic function tests: Cholinergic receptors: Muscarinic receptors*

Australian Therapeutic Trial in Mild Hypertension (Lancet (1980) 1:1261-1267)

This trial was a single blind study comparing antihypertensive treatment (n=1721) to placebo treatment (n=1706) for an average of four years in subjects aged 30-69 years.

Active treatment consisted of step-wise addition of chlorothiazide, methyldopa, propranolol or pindolol and hydralazine or clonidine, aiming to reduce diastolic blood pressure to, for instance, less than or equal to 90 mmHg.

The study showed that drug treatment for patients with diastolic pressures in the range 95-109 mmHg without end-organ damage will reduce cardiovascular mortality and morbidity significantly. The main effect was on cerebrovascular disease. Events related to ischaemic heart disease were reduced by treatment, but not significantly. It is necessary to treat large numbers to benefit a few, however. For example, approximately one death was prevented per 500 patient years of treatment. See also *Multi-centre studies of clinical outcome*

Autacoid

A local hormone. This term embraces substances as diverse as histamine, 5-hydroxytryptamine, angiotensins, kinins and prostaglandins.

Autonomic function tests

A number of tests are available to study the function of the autonomic nervous system. They are used particularly in the investigation of patients with evidence of autonomic neuropathies and/or orthostatic (postural) hypotension.

Tests predominantly of sympathetic function include:

Blood pressure response to sustained handgrip

Autonomic function tests

Maximum voluntary contraction (MVC) is first determined by asking the patient to squeeze a rolled sphygmomanometer cuff as tightly as possible and taking the highest reading of three on the manometer. Handgrip is then maintained at 30% MVC for as long as possible up to five minutes. Blood pressure is measured in the opposite arm three times before and at one minute intervals during handgrip. Results (highest diastolic pressure during handgrip minus mean of diastolic readings before) are:-
> normal ⩾16 mmHg;
> borderline 11-15 mmHg;
> abnormal ⩽10 mmHg.

This is a test for the sharp rise in blood pressure which normally occurs with sustained handgrip due to increased cardiac output and heart rate.

Blood pressure response to standing
Supine blood pressure is recorded after ten minutes rest. The patient then stands briskly and erect blood pressure is recorded at 30 seconds, one minute and two minutes. Systolic blood pressure should not fall by much more than 15 mmHg. More than 20 mmHg is regarded as clearly abnormal. In a normal patient pooling of blood in the legs on standing is rapidly corrected by peripheral vasoconstriction, hence blood pressure does not fall dramatically.

Cold-pressor test
see *Cold pressor test*
Tests predominantly of parasympathetic function include:
> *Heart rate response to Valsalva manoeuvre*
see *Valsalva manoeuvre*
> *Immediate heart rate response to standing*

The patient lies quietly while the electrocardiogram (ECG) is recorded continuously, so that heart rate can be assessed by measuring the R-R interval. The patient then stands up and the corresponding point is marked on the ECG tracing. Response is quoted as a 30:15 ratio, that is

$$\frac{\text{Longest R-R interval at or around 30th beat after standing}}{\text{Shortest R-R interval at or around 15th beat after standing}}$$

Results (in terms of the 30:15 ratio) are:
> normal ⩾1.04;
> borderline 1.01-1.03;
> abnormal ⩽1.00.

This test depends on a vagally mediated overshoot slowing of the pulse maximal around beat 30 which normally follows the immediate increase in heart rate with standing.

> *Heart rate variation during deep breathing*

The patient sits quietly and breathes deeply at six breaths per minute (five seconds inspiration, then five seconds expiration) for one minute. The ECG is recorded and the onset of each inspiration and expiration is marked on the tracing. Maximum and minimum R-R intervals during each respiratory cycle are measured and converted to beats per minute. The results (mean of the differences between maximum and minimum heart rates for the six cycles in beats/minute) are:
> normal ⩾15;
> borderline 11-14;
> abnormal ⩽10.

This test depends on the fact that normal variation in heart rate with respiration requires an intact parasympathetic nerve supply.

Abnormalities of sympathetic function
These often present with syncope and/or postural hypotension without an appropriate heart rate response. It may be useful to separate the preganglionic lesions (a central fault in which the lateral horn cells of the thoracic spinal cord degenerate) from the postganglionic lesions (in which neurones of ganglia degenerate).

Preganglionic form In the preganglionic form, resting circulating concentrations of noradrenaline tend to be near normal but do not rise appropriately on standing;

the blood pressure response to infused noradrenaline or alpha-agonists like phenylephrine is normal.

Postganglionic form In the postganglionic type, noradrenaline is not released normally and therefore circulating noradrenaline concentrations are low leading to hypersensitivity of the blood pressure response to injected exogenous noradrenaline or alpha-agonists like phenylephrine; again circulating concentrations fail to rise when the subject stands.

Characteristics The preganglionic type have intact postganglionic nerve endings, therefore intravenous infusion of tyramine will cause release of noradrenaline from these, thus raising blood pressure to a similar extent to that observed when tyramine is given to a normal subject. Infusion of tyramine may also cause pressure to rise in those with postganglionic lesions because, although tyramine is not now able to release noradrenaline from peripheral nerve endings (which have degenerated), the postsynaptic sites are supersensitive, having been exposed to very low circulating noradrenaline concentrations, and tyramine's direct sympathomimetic action may now be able to manifest itself. However, the response to tyramine is usually less marked than in normals or those with the central types of lesions.

Abnormalities of parasympathetic function
If the tests of parasympathetic function are abnormal further information may be obtained by studying the response to intravenous atropine. A dose of 0.03 mg/kg injected over three minutes normally produces an increase of at least 20 beats per minute at some time during 10 further minutes. If the parasympathetic tests are abnormal, a normal atropine test implies an afferent lesion and a blunted atropine response could be due to either an afferent or efferent lesion.

Other tests of autonomic function
These include sweat tests, measurements of plasma renin and noradrenaline concentrations before and after tilting on a tilt table, and tests of the pupillary response to various drugs. Results of the tests may be difficult to interpret in the elderly as ageing may cause changes which require to be distinguished from those related to a specific disease process. Some of the tests may be hazardous (for example, tilting), particularly to elderly patients. See also *Orthostatic hypotension*

Autonomic nervous system
The system comprising the autonomic ganglia and nerves concerned with control of the internal environment.
This control is achieved by innervation of the non-skeletal muscle of the heart, blood vessels, bronchial tree, gut and pupils, and by the secretomotor supply of many glands including those of the gut and its outgrowths, the sweat glands and the adrenal medulla. Afferent fibres arise from visceral organs, skin and great vessels and carry information to the central nervous system (CNS) where the data are integrated. The efferent fibres, which supply the organs and tissues detailed above, carry the output of the sympathetic and parasympathetic nervous systems. A unique feature is the fact that the autonomic (sympathetic or para-sympathetic) fibres that leave the CNS terminate in ganglia (preganglionic neurones). The postganglionic neurone, which synapses with the preganglionic neurone, then proceeds to the organ or tissue supplied. See also *Central nervous system: Parasympathetic nervous system: Sympathetic nervous system*

Autonomic reflex
Reflex mediated by components of the autonomic nervous system.

Autoregulation of blood flow
Intrinsic capacity of tissues to control their own blood flow in response to changes in perfusion pressure. In response

Autoregulation of blood flow

to increased pressure, vessels constrict,
preventing or reducing an increase in flow.
Well-developed in the kidney, but also
seen in mesentery, skeletal muscles, brain,
liver and myocardium. See also *Cerebral
circulation*

AV3V
see *Anteroventral third ventricle*

Azamethonium bromide
A ganglion-blocking antihypertensive
agent.

Azotaemia
Renal failure.

B

Bainbridge reflex
(Francis Arthur Bainbridge, English physiologist, 1874-1921)
A rise in heart rate of anaesthetized animals sometimes produced by rapid infusion of blood or saline.
It appears to be a true reflex, rather than a response to local stretch, since infusion of fluids in animals with transplanted hearts increases the rate of the recipient's atrial remnant, but fails to affect the rate of the transplanted heart. The effect is blocked by atropine and diminished or absent when the initial heart rate is high, indicating that it is mediated by the vagus nerve. The effect is of uncertain physiological significance.

Ballistocardiogram
Tracing recorded by a ballistocardiograph.

Ballistocardiograph
A device for recording the movements of the body caused by the cardiac impulse, which is used to determine the degree of elasticity of the aorta and to calculate cardiac output.

Balloon angioplasty
see *Angioplasty*

Baroreceptors
Baroreceptors are sensory nerve endings which act as stretch receptors and thereby detect changes in blood pressure within the heart and blood vessels.
These receptors are found in the carotid sinus, the aortic arch, the heart, and the pulmonary circulation. They discharge nerve impulses at an increased rate in response to increased pressure. Afferent nerve fibres in the vagus nerve and the glossopharyngeal nerve relay the information to the medulla. Most of these fibres terminate in a structure called the nucleus of the tractus solitarius (NTS), though some pass directly to the cardio-

inhibitory centre. As the afferent fibres synapse with inhibitory interneurones in the NTS, activation of these interneurones (resulting from increased discharge in the afferent fibres) leads to inhibition of the vasomotor centre (Figure 19). Decreased output from the vasomotor centre, in the efferent nerve fibres, then leads to vasodilatation and a fall in blood pressure. See also *Arterial baroreceptors: Cardiac baroreceptors: Cardiopulmonary receptors*

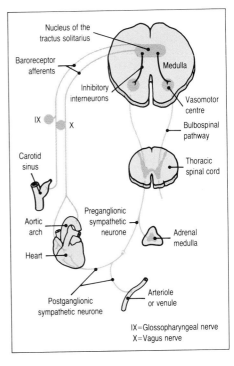

Figure 19 Baroreceptors. Diagram to show the baroreceptors, their afferent nerve supply (red), the vasomotor centre, and the efferent pathway (green)

Baroreceptors and hypertension
(special contribution from Professor Thomas G. Pickering, The New York Hospital-Cornell Medical Center, New York, USA)

Baroreceptors and hypertension

Baroreceptors are pressure-sensitive sensory receptors located in the walls of the arteries and heart, which play an important role in the reflex regulation of the circulation. They can be conveniently divided into high pressure and low pressure receptors.

High pressure baroreceptors
High pressure receptors are located mainly in the aortic arch and carotid sinus; they respond both to dynamic and static components of pressure. Stimulation by an increase of pressure results in a reflex slowing of the heart and vasodilatation. Their major role is probably in buffering acute changes of blood pressure rather than in its long-term regulation.

In hypertension, the baroreceptors are reset to the higher level of pressure, that is, the firing rate in the afferent nerves is normal, so that the baroreflex operates to maintain the pressure at that level. The sensitivity of the baroreflex may be measured by comparing the reflex response (for example, change of heart rate) to the stimulus (for instance, drug-induced change of arterial pressure, or change of transmural pressure in the carotid sinus produced by neck suction). It is diminished both by hypertension and ageing. Both resetting and the loss of sensitivity may be mediated by changes in the physical properties of the arterial wall.

Low pressure baroreceptors
The low pressure receptors are located in the walls of the atria, ventricles and pulmonary vessels, and respond to changes in cardiac filling pressure such as occur during postural changes or haemorrhage.

The afferent nerves are probably the vagi. The reflex response to a decreased filling pressure (which can be produced experimentally by lower body negative pressure, causing pooling of blood in the legs) is a vasoconstriction and increased renin secretion. In contrast to the diminished sensitivity of the high pressure reflexes, this reflex response appears to be augmented in patients with mild hypertension, and it is also preserved with ageing.

Renal baroreceptors
These receptors have also been postulated as one of the mediators of renin release by the kidney.

They are most probably situated in the afferent arterioles of the glomeruli, and respond to decreased stretch (as in hypotension) by augmenting renin release. This may be mediated by changes in the synthesis of renal prostaglandins rather than by a reflex mechanism. There are also afferent nerves from the kidney which produce reflex effects, but their role in clinical hypertension is unknown. See also *Baroreceptors*

Bartter's syndrome

(Frederic Crosby Bartter, U.S. physiologist, born 1914-1983)
A disease characterized by hypokalaemia secondary to renal potassium wasting, metabolic alkalosis, elevated plasma levels of renin and aldosterone with resistance to the pressor effect of exogenous angiotensin II, hyperplasia of the renal juxtaglomerular apparatus, normal blood pressure and the absence of oedema. Children may present with growth retardation and adults with symptoms of hypokalaemia (for instance, polyuria, muscular weakness).

Differential diagnosis includes surreptitious diuretic or purgative abuse and secret vomiting. Treatment is unsatisfactory but there is often a good response to cyclooxygenase inhibitors such as indomethacin.

Basal arterial pressure

Arterial pressure recorded with the patient in a rested, relaxed state. To achieve this it is necessary to habituate the patients to blood pressure measurement and, according to some workers, rest them overnight.

Bendrofluazide

see *Thiazide diuretics*

Bendroflumethiazide
Synonym for bendrofluazide.

Benign hypertension
Term used to denote hypertension without features of the malignant phase hypertension. Although benign hypertension may be mild, the term should probably be avoided as patients with mild hypertension are nevertheless at increased risk of cardiovascular damage. See also *Arterial hypertension: Complications of hypertension*

Benzothiazides
Synonym for bendrofluazide.

Benzthiazide
see *Thiazide diuretics*

Benzydroflumethiazide
see *Thiazide diuretics*

Beriberi
Syndrome caused by thiamine deficiency. Hypertension may appear transiently during its treatment.

Berry aneurysms
Small saccular aneurysms of a cerebral artery usually seen on the Circle of Willis and its major branches (Figure 20). Often found at points of bifurcation, and possibly resulting from congenital defects. Development of berry aneurysms may be associated with hypertension and diffuse arteriosclerosis. They are also more common in patients with coarctation of the aorta or polycystic kidneys. The rupture of a berry aneurysm is the commonest cause of subarachnoid haemorrhage.

Beta-adrenergic receptor blocking drugs
These drugs are antagonists which bind to beta-adrenergic receptors (Table 7). Like the thiazide diuretics, they are regarded as first line therapy for hypertension because of their safety, tolerability and efficacy. Beta-blockers are also useful in the treatment of angina pectoris and for the secondary prevention of myocardial infarction. Their precise mechanism of action in lowering blood

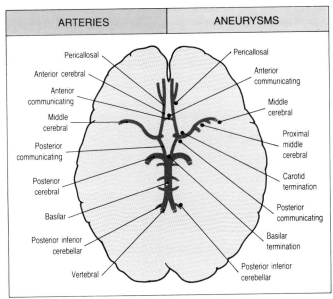

ARTERIES	ANEURYSMS

Pericallosal
Anterior cerebral
Anterior communicating
Middle cerebral
Posterior communicating
Posterior cerebral
Basilar
Posterior inferior cerebellar
Vertebral

Pericallosal
Anterior communicating
Middle cerebral
Proximal middle cerebral
Carotid termination
Posterior communicating
Basilar termination
Posterior inferior cerebellar

Figure 20
Berry aneurysms. Common sites of aneurysms on the Circle of Willis

Beta-adrenergic receptor blocking drugs

Table 7 Beta-adrenergic receptor blocking drugs

Drug	Cardio-selectivity	Partial agonist activity	Elimination half life (h)	Usual dosage frequency[1]
(A) Cardioselective				
(1) Atenolol	+	0	6-9	od / bd
(2) Metoprolol	+	0	3-4	od / bd [2]
(3) Acebutolol	±	+	8*	od / bd
(B) Non-selective				
(1) Pindolol	0	+++	3-4	bd /tds
(2) Oxprenolol	0	++	2	bd [2]
(3) Timolol	0	±	4-5	od / bd
(4) Propranolol	0	0	3.5-6	bd [2]
(5) Sotalol	0	0	13-17	od / bd
(6) Nadolol	0	0	17-24	od

od=once daily ; bd= twice daily; tds= thrice daily;
* Acebutolol is converted to active metabolite diacetolol on passage through the liver; half life combines both compounds
1 Recommended for Hypertension in British National Formulary
2 Sustained release preparations available designed for once daily administration

pressure is obscure, but may include reduction of cardiac output, suppression of renin, and central effects. Those which are relatively specific for the $beta_1$-receptor are described as cardioselective (for example, atenolol, metoprolol) and are less likely than non-cardioselective beta blockers (like propranolol) to worsen airways obstruction in asthmatics. Neither group of drugs should, however, be used in these patients.

Beta blockers with intrinsic sympatho-mimetic (partial agonist) activity (such as pindolol) cause less bradycardia and may even increase resting heart rate. Side-effects of beta blockers include worsening of cardiac failure, worsening of intermittent claudication, lethargy and CNS effects which include vivid dreams and, rarely, depression. See also *Beta-adrenergic receptors*

Beta-adrenergic receptors
Beta-adrenergic receptors were differentiated from alpha-adrenergic receptors by studying the relative potencies of various adrenergic agonists (*see* Table 1).

The use of more specific drugs allowed the beta-receptors to be divided into $beta_1$ and $beta_2$ subtypes. Of the beta-adrenergic receptor blocking drugs, metoprolol and practolol are the agents *in vitro* with the greatest specificity for the $beta_1$-receptor (although atenolol appears more cardioselective than metoprolol *in vivo*). *In vitro* the potency of metoprolol in blocking the $beta_1$-receptor is about twenty times its potency at the $beta_2$-receptor. $beta_1$-receptors are postsynaptic, whereas $beta_2$-receptors as well as being postsynaptic may be presynaptic (stimulation facilitates noradrenaline release from the nerve ending) and nonsynaptic (for example, on white blood cells).

Both receptor subtypes trigger intracellular events by interacting with guanine nucleotide binding proteins and stimulating adenylate cyclase. Beta-adrenergic receptors have been identified and characterized on many tissues by using radioactively labelled antagonists with high specific activity, for example, iodopindolol. The receptor proteins from various sources have been purified by affinity chromatography. The receptor is a single glycosylated polypeptide, the molecular weight of which varies depending on the source. It is possible to reconstitute the purified receptor in membranes with the components of the adenylate cyclase system. See also *Alpha-adrenergic receptors: Beta-adrenergic receptor blocking drugs*

Beta-lipotrophin (β-LPH)
see *Pro-opiomelanocortin*

Bethanidine
Adrenergic neurone blocking agent with a shorter duration of action than guanethidine, and is not commonly prescribed because of frequency of postural hypotension and impotence. See also *Adrenergic neurone blocking agents*

Bianchi-Milan spontaneously hypertensive rats
(Guiseppe Bianchi, Italian physician) Strain of rats bred to develop hypertension and used as a model for its experimental study. The cause of hypertension is thought to lie within the kidney. See *Dahl rats: Okamoto strain of spontaneously hypertensive rat: Rat strains in hypertension research*

Bicuculline
A gamma-aminobutyrate (GABA) antagonist. Central administration of this drug in some experimental animals increases blood pressure, possibly implicating GABA in central blood pressure regulation.

Big renin
(*also known as* Big inactive renin) see *Inactive renin: Renin*

Bilateral aldosteronism
Primary aldosteronism with over-

production of the hormone by both adrenal glands.
Bilateral aldosteronism is almost always due to bilateral adrenocortical hyperplasia. Cases of bilateral aldosteronomas have been reported, but some of these may represent the coexistence of an aldosteronoma in one adrenal with a non-functioning adenoma (adrenocortical nodule) in the other. See also *Conn's syndrome: Idiopathic aldosteronism*

Bilateral nephrectomy
Blood pressure may be difficult to control in some patients with chronic renal failure undergoing dialysis or with a transplanted kidney because of secretion of renin from the residual kidneys. Removal of both remaining kidneys to control pressure (Figure 21) has been superseded by use of converting enzyme inhibitors to prevent formation of the active peptide angiotensin II by the action of the enzyme renin on its substrate. See also *Angiotensin I converting enzyme inhibitors: Dialysis*

Biofeedback
Techniques of self-induced relaxation to lower blood pressure.

Blaustein hypothesis
(Mordecai P Blaustein, born 1935, U.S. physiologist)
It has been suggested by various groups that intracellular sodium is increased in essential hypertension. Some workers have postulated the existence of a 'natriuretic hormone' which might cause increased intracellular sodium by inhibiting the Na^+-K^+ pump.
Blaustein pointed out that inhibition of calcium-sodium exchange by either increased intracellular sodium or decreased extracellular sodium would produce increased intracellular calcium. When cytosolic calcium concentration lies within a critical range, Blaustein calculated that smooth muscle tension would be critically dependent on intracellular sodium concentration.

Blaustein hypothesis

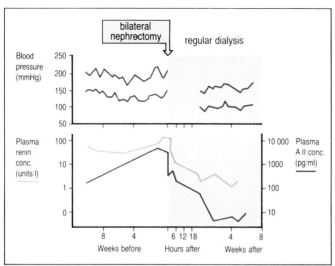

Figure 21 Bilateral nephrectomy. Bilateral nephrectomy in a patient on dialysis with high renin levels: effects on blood pressure plasma renin concentration and plasma angiotensin II concentration

A 5% increase in intracellular sodium concentration might increase smooth muscle tension by about 50%. It should be stressed that the Blaustein hypothesis does not necessarily require that the increased intracellular sodium is caused by the putative natriuretic hormone. See also *Calcium: Calcium sodium exchange*

Blockade
Binding of an antagonist to a receptor causes blockade of that receptor. See also *Antagonist: Receptors*

Blood-brain barrier
The barrier separating the blood from the parenchyma of the central nervous system.
It probably consists of the capillary walls and the adjacent glial membranes. The ability of drugs to cross the blood-brain barrier may influence their effects (beneficial and adverse). The circum-ventricular organs lie outwith the blood-brain barrier.

Blood flow
Distribution of the cardiac output to the various parts of the body.
For a 63 kg man with a mean arterial pressure of 90 mmHg, mean cardiac output is 5400 ml/min. (Table 8)

Table 8 Distribution of blood flow

	ml/min.
Liver	1500
Kidney	1260
Brain	750
Skin	462
Skeletal muscle	840
Heart muscle	250
Rest of body	336

These figures reflect distribution at rest and alter with exercise

Blood pressure
see *Arterial blood pressure*

Blood screening tests

Measurements of serum concentrations of urea, creatinine and electrolytes are extensively used as screening tests in hypertensive patients. Hypokalaemia with increased serum concentrations of bicarbonate and sodium may be the first indication of primary aldosteronism (or other forms of mineralocorticoid hypertension, including 17α-hydroxylase deficiency, carbenoxolone or liquorice ingestion). With secondary aldosteronism, for example, in malignant phase hypertension, hypokalaemia is generally accompanied by low normal or low serum sodium concentration. Thiazide diuretics may also cause hypokalaemia. Raised concentrations of urea and creatinine may indicate renal damage due to severe hypertension or primary renal disease causing hypertension.

Blood tests in hypertension evaluation

Measurement of substances in the blood is often essential in the diagnosis of the cause of secondary hypertension. In primary aldosteronism, high plasma aldosterone concentrations are associated with suppression of plasma renin activity. In cases due to an aldosteronoma, adrenal vein sampling will reliably indicate the side of the lesion. Blood tests are also essential in the diagnosis of other endocrine causes of hypertension, for example, Cushing's syndrome and phaeochromocytoma. In renal hypertension, including renal artery stenosis, peripheral blood concentrations of renin and angiotensin II may be high. The measurements of renin in samples of blood from the renal veins will indicate the kidney from which excessive renin is being secreted in patients with unilateral renal artery stenosis. The predictive value of this test in selecting patients for corrective surgery is still controversial.

Blood vessel walls

see *Arterial wall*

Blood volume

Total blood volume is given by multiplying plasma volume by 100/(100-haematocrit) where haematocrit is quoted as a percentage.

Plasma volume can be measured using dyes, for example, Evans Blue, which bind to plasma proteins, or by the use of albumin labelled with radioactive iodine. Average plasma volume is 3500 ml for a 70 kg man. Red cell volume is given by subtracting plasma volume from total blood volume, or it can be measured by the dilution of red blood cells labelled with radioactive isotopes, for example ^{51}Chromium.

Blood and plasma volumes appear to be reduced in men with essential hypertension whether they are of normal weight or obese. In women the volumes are found, on average, to be normal. See *Haematocrit*

Body fat

see *Body mass index: Obesity and hypertension*

Body mass index (BMI)

Measurement of obesity obtained by dividing weight in kilograms by height squared where height is measured in metres. It correlates well with body fat. Life insurance statistics show a significant increase in mortality when BMI is above 30. See also *Obesity and hypertension*

Body potassium

see *Body sodium and potassium*

Body sodium and potassium

Total body sodium (TBNa) can be determined by whole body counting after *in vivo* activation of sodium by neutron bombardment. Body sodium is distributed as follows: 40% in bone, 55% extracellular, 5% intracellular.

Total body potassium (TBK) can be determined by measuring the naturally-occurring isotope ^{40}K using a whole body

Body sodium and potassium

counter. In order to make comparisons of body sodium and body potassium between subjects it is necessary to correct for variation in size and shape. Mean values for TBNa, TBK and exchangeable sodium and potassium (Na_E and K_E) are normal in untreated essential hypertension. However, unlike the situation in normals, TBNa and Na_E are positively, and TBK and K_E negatively related to both systolic and diastolic pressure.

The positive relationship with sodium is most marked with more severe hypertension, and in older patients. It has been postulated that in early essential hypertension blood pressure is raised by a mechanism not involving sodium retention. Later, sodium retention may become important, perhaps resulting from renal changes secondary to hypertension. See also *Exchangeable sodium and potassium*

Body surface area nomogram
Device for estimating body surface area from measurements of height and weight. Allows, for example, a measurement of creatinine clearance to be compared with the normal for age and sex quoted per 1.73 m^2.

Body weight
see *Body mass index: Obesity and hypertension*

Bolometer
Device for measuring the force of cardiac contraction.

Bombesin
A tetradecapeptide isolated from the skin of the frog *Bombina bombina*, which has spasmogenic activity in a variety of vascular and non-vascular smooth muscle structures.

It causes vasoconstriction and hypertension in most animal species, but not in man. A mammalian counterpart, with 27 amino acid residues, called gastrin-releasing peptide has been found in the brain and gastrointestinal tract.

Borderline hypertension
This is the condition in which a patient's blood pressure is above the normal range but not sufficiently high to merit antihypertensive treatment. It is common. One study found that 23% of individuals tested over a three-week period had borderline diastolic readings. Diastolic borderline hypertension is less common than systolic. Many studies suggest that patients with borderline hypertension are more than twice as likely as normotensive individuals to develop subsequent established hypertension emphasizing the need for careful follow-up of such patients (Figure 22). Having said this, however, the majority of borderline hypertensives do not become established hypertensives.

Many studies indicate that patients with borderline hypertension are at increased risk of cardiovascular morbidity and mortality compared with normotensive controls. The pathogenesis of borderline hypertension is unclear. Individuals with this condition may have increased activity of the sympathetic nervous system, and possibly also decreased activity of the parasympathetic nervous system. See also *Arterial hypertension: Labile hypertension*

Bothrops jararaca venom
Venom from this Brazilian viper was the source of the first series of peptides found to enhance bradykinin's action and later to inhibit angiotensin-converting enzyme, leading to the development of the orally active converting enzyme inhibitors for use in the treatment of hypertension.

Bouchard-Charcot microaneurysms
(Charles Jacques Bouchard, French physician, 1837-1915; Jean-Martin Charcot, French neurologist, 1825-1893)
These tiny aneurysms affect the small intracerebral arteries 50-150 μm in

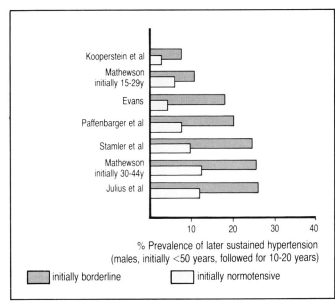

Figure 22 Borderline hypertension. Prevalence of later sustained hypertension in patients who were initially either normotensive or borderline hypertensive. The prevalence in initially borderline patients is consistently higher than that for initially normotensive patients

% Prevalence of later sustained hypertension
(males, initially <50 years, followed for 10-20 years)

☐ initially borderline   ☐ initially normotensive

diameter. They are caused by replacement of the lining endothelium, media and elastic tissue by fibrous tissue, and are more common in hypertensive patients. Rupture of these microaneurysms results in intracerebral haemorrhage. See also *Aneurysm: Arterial wall: Cerebral haemorrhage*

Bowman's space
(Sir William Bowman, English ophthalmologist, anatomist and physiologist, 1816-1892)
The space within Bowman's capsule which is the dilated blind end of the nephron. The glomerular tuft of capillaries protrudes into the side of the Bowman's capsule. Blood in the glomerular capillary is thus separated from Bowman's space by a thin layer of tissue composed of the single-celled capillary lining, the basement membrane and the single-celled lining of Bowman's capsule. This allows filtration of fluid from the capillaries into Bowman's space. See also *Glomerulus: Nephron*

Bradycardia
A heart rate arbitrarily of less than 60 beats per minute.
Beta-adrenergic receptor blockers commonly cause bradycardia by blocking cardiac beta₁-receptors. Beta-blockers with intrinsic sympathomimetic activity (for example, pindolol) cause less reduction in heart rate, but bradycardia with beta-blockers is rarely of clinical significance. See also *Beta-adrenergic receptor blocking drugs: Cardiac rate*

Bradycrotic
Pertaining to, or causing, bradycardia.

Bradykinin
A nonapeptide member of the kinin group of autocoids that is produced by the action of plasma kallikrein on high molecular weight kininogen (HMWK).
Both bradykinin and kallidin have similar effects on the cardiovascular system, extravascular smooth muscle, and nervous tissue. See also *Kallikreins: Kinins*

Bradysphygmia
Synonym for bradycardia.

Brain angiotensinogen
Angiotensinogen is present in cerebrospinal fluid and in brain tissue. Highest concentrations are found in the area postrema, the organum vasculosum of the lamina terminalis, the periventricular region of the thalamus and hypothalamus and the median eminence. See also *Angiotensins: Brain renin-angiotensin system: Circumventricular organs*

Brain angiotensins
Angiotensin I has been found in human, dog and rat cerebrospinal fluid (CSF) as well as brain tissue. Angiotensin II is also found in CSF, as is angiotensin III. Most of the angiotensin-like immunoreactivity in the brain is in nerve endings rather than cell bodies, but staining in cell bodies can be enhanced with colchicine. Staining is largely in the cell bodies of the supraoptic and paraventricular neurones which secrete antidiuretic hormone. In endings staining has a different distribution, but a pathway can be identified from the paraventricular nucleus to the median eminence. See also *Brain renin-angiotensin system*

Brain converting enzyme
Small, but measurable amounts of converting enzyme are found in the cerebrospinal fluid. Brain tissue contains larger amounts with highest converting enzyme concentrations in the locus ceruleus, substantia nigra and hypothalamus. See also *Angiotensin I converting enzyme: Brain renin-angiotensin system*

Brain peptides and blood pressure control (special contribution from Dr D. Ganten, Deutsches Institut zur Bekämpfung des hohen Blutdruckes, Heidelberg, Germany)
Immunohistochemical and biochemical investigations have revealed numerous peptides within the brain. Evidence has been obtained supporting a role in blood pressure regulation for centrally located angiotensin, opioid peptides, substance P, neuropeptide Y, antidiuretic hormone, atrial natriuretic peptide (ANP), kinins, corticotrophin releasing factor and other peptides, such as bombesin and somatostatin.

Angiotensin II
The effector peptide of the renin-angiotensin system, angiotensin II has been found by immunohistochemical and molecular biological techniques to be present in the brain (Figure 23). The central actions of angiotensin II have been studied by, firstly, administering the peptide exogenously to the brain ventricular system, secondly, by topical application to angiotensin II-sensitive sites located around the brain ventricles or, thirdly, by stimulating the synthesis of endogenous angiotensin II through the injection of renin into the brain ventricles. Using this latter procedure, the injected renin cleaves the decapeptide angiotensin I from the high molecular weight precursor angiotensinogen and, by the action of brain converting enzyme, the octapeptide angiotensin II, is generated. Angiotensin II can then activate specific receptors in the brain leading to characteristic cardiovascular, behavioural and neurohumoral effects, namely, an increase in blood pressure, stimulation of salt and water intake, and release of the antidiuretic hormone (ADH) and oxytocin from the hypothalamus and adrenocorticotropic hormone (ACTH) from the pituitary gland. In addition, increases in plasma noradrenaline and adrenaline and a marked natriuretic effect have been observed. These central effects of angiotensin II can (with the exception of natriuresis) also be produced by circulating angiotensin II acting directly on central sites outside the blood-brain barrier, which the peptide cannot cross freely. Brain sites sensitive to circulating

angiotensin II are the subfornical organ, the organum vasculosum laminae terminalis (OVLT) and the area postrema. Evidence for a pathophysiological role of brain angiotensin in the maintenance of high blood pressure has mainly been gathered in the spontaneously hypertensive rat. In these animals, increased renin levels have been observed in blood pressure controlling brain areas during the development of hypertension, and the intracerebroventricular administration of specific inhibitors of the brain renin-angiotensin system has been found to lower the elevated blood pressure.

Opioid peptides

Endorphins, dynorphins, encephalins are widely distributed throughout the central nervous system. The occurrence of both short-chain encephalins and endorphins in the hypothalamus and encephalins, endorphins and dynorphins in the nucleus of the tractus solitarius (NTS) points towards a participation in central cardiovascular control.

The pentapeptide encephalins seem to be pressor when administered to the brain ventricular system of conscious dogs, cats and rats, but can also induce depressor effects in anaesthetized animals. In contrast, the long-chain opioid peptides, such as beta-endorphin, appear to be mainly depressor. The vagal component of the baroreceptor reflex can be markedly attenuated by central encephalin treatment. See also *Opioid peptides*

Substance P

This is an undecapeptide with a wide distribution within the peripheral and central nervous systems, particularly high

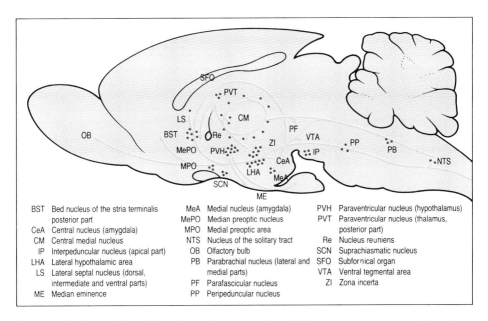

BST	Bed nucleus of the stria terminalis, posterior part	MeA	Medial nucleus (amygdala)	PVH	Paraventricular nucleus (hypothalamus)
CeA	Central nucleus (amygdala)	MePO	Median preoptic nucleus	PVT	Paraventricular nucleus (thalamus, posterior part)
CM	Central medial nucleus	MPO	Medial preoptic area	Re	Nucleus reuniens
IP	Interpeduncular nucleus (apical part)	NTS	Nucleus of the solitary tract	SCN	Suprachiasmatic nucleus
LHA	Lateral hypothalamic area	OB	Olfactory bulb	SFO	Subfornical organ
LS	Lateral septal nucleus (dorsal, intermediate and ventral parts)	PB	Parabrachial nucleus (lateral and medial parts)	VTA	Ventral tegmental area
ME	Median eminence	PF	Parafascicular nucleus	ZI	Zona incerta
		PP	Peripeduncular nucleus		

Figure 23 **Brain peptides**. This schematic mid-sagittal view of the rat brain illustrates the major angiotensin II immunoreactive cell groups and fibre systems. Arrowheads are drawn to indicate the orientation of projections. Note that angiotensin II-stained cells and fibres are most prominent in regions that have been implicated in the behavioural, autonomic, and endocrine control of the homeostasis, indicating that angiotensin II may play an especially important role in central systems involved in fluid balance

Brain peptides and blood pressure

concentrations being present in the hypothalamus. Like bradykinin, it has potent depressor effects when applied peripherally, but has marked pressor activity when administered to the brain ventricular system in both conscious and anaesthetized animals. See also *Bradykinin*

Corticotrophin releasing factor (CRF)
CRF apparently participates in the integration of cardiovascular and humoral responses to different kinds of stress. CRF has been localized in a number of hypothalamic and extrahypothalamic nuclei, including the limbic system and the medulla oblongata.

Apart from releasing ACTH and beta-endorphin from the pituitary, it also increases blood pressure by increasing sympathetic tone. Humoral and neuronal pathways are thus activated to achieve a concerted cardiovascular response to stress. See also *ACTH: Corticotrophin releasing factor*

Antidiuretic hormone (ADH)
This is instrumental in fluid and volume homeostasis and, like angiotensin, seems to exert its effects both centrally and peripherally. However, its central actions may be even more complex than those of angiotensin II, activating both blood pressure increasing pathways and blood pressure lowering pathways. This may be explained by the fact that ADH can be stimulated by iso-osmotic hypovolaemia as well as by normo- or hypervolaemic hyper-osmolality.

In the first case (for example, following haemorrhage) an antidiuretic and pressor action of ADH would be logical in order to regain volume homeostasis and to improve the haemodynamic situation.

In the second case (for example, salt loading) a depressor action together with renal water reabsorption might be the more adequate response, since there is no volume deficit and blood pressure may be normal or possibly increased.

Mode of peptide action
The neuropeptides constitute such a large and diverse group of compounds that no meaningful generalization concerning their mode of action can be made. Nevertheless, there are certain features which should be stressed in this context.

Neuropeptides have been found to coexist with each other or with monoamine transmitters, thereby greatly increasing the variety of chemical signals that a neurone can utilize when communicating with other cells. If these transmitters are packaged together within a single vesicle of the neurone terminal, it is possible that a synaptic 'cocktail', consisting of peptides, monoamines and amino acids can be simultaneously released. However, each transmitter may also be released separately.

In general, peptide effects occur over a longer time course and over greater distances ('neuro-hormonal' action) than is the case for other neurotransmitters. Fundamental differences exist between biogenic amines, amino acids and peptides in their modes of synthesis and meta-bolism. In particular, peptides are not as rapidly degraded as the classic transmitters and are also probably not recycled. These differences in the rate of synthesis, transport and replenishment of transmitter allows the possibility that similar repetitive stimuli may elicit quite different postsynaptic patterns in pepti-dergic as opposed to non-peptidergic neurones.

All peptides are synthesized as high molecular weight precursors. Several active peptides can be released by enzymatic cleavage from one precursor and act at different receptors. These 'peptide families' can bring about a number of different actions, which in most instances appear to be teleologically meaningful. Since these 'concerted action' peptides originate from, and are controlled and regulated by, one single gene, they may comprise actions on heart and kidney function, on the autonomic nervous system activity and on hormone release but also on such complex behaviours as pain perception, salt appetite, drinking and feeding. Since several forms of cardio-vascular disease are caused by health damaging behaviour patterns,it is tempting to speculate that peptides may provide a clue to the better understanding of this behavioural aspect at a molecular level. The relevance of these factors for cardiovascular control remains to be established. Nevertheless, the functional subdivision of the autonomic nervous system according to the co-localization of peptides has certainly opened exciting new avenues for both the understanding and possibly the treatment of hypertensive disease.

Summary
These peptides have been localized in brain areas known to be important in cardiovascular control.
Specific high-affinity peptide receptors have been discovered in the brain.
Upon central administration the peptides produce blood pressure effects, which can be prevented by competitive antagonists and they interact with other blood pressure-controlling neuroregulators, for example, catecholamines or gamma-aminobutyrate (GABA).
Central inhibition of brain peptide synthesis or interaction with brain peptide receptors results in marked cardiovascular effects.
Peptide levels and the activity of synthesizing enzymes are altered in hypertensive states.
Supersensitivity to the pressor action of some brain peptides in experimental models of hypertension has been described.
See also *Atrial natriuretic peptides: Bombesin: Brain renin-angiotensin system: Central neurotransmitters: Kinins: Neuropeptides: Somatostatin*

Brain renin
Brain renin activity has been demonstrated by incubating angiotensinogen with brain tissue at low pH. There is good evidence that at least some of the angiotensin I generation is catalyzed by renin and not by cathepsin D. Highest amounts appear to be in the pineal gland, the anterior pituitary and the choroid plexus. Brain renin differs slightly from that in the kidney in terms of molecular weight and isoelectric point. See also *Aspartyl proteases: Brain renin-angiotensin system: Renin*

Brain renin-angiotensin system
All the components of the renin-angiotensin system, including angiotensin II receptors, are present in the central nervous system. Under usual conditions, these substances are not of peripheral origin and are thought to be synthesized in the brain. The effects of intracerebro-ventricular angiotensin II that are also produced by intravenous angiotensin II (for instance, increased drinking, increased blood pressure, and increased secretion of ADH) are probably due to angiotensin II in the cerebrospinal fluid penetrating the circumventricular organs. The brain renin-angiotensin system may alter output of monoamines from nor-adrenergic and dopaminergic neurones in the brain. The reported effects on blood pressure in hypertensive animals could be exerted via central adrenergic systems. See also *Brain peptides and blood pressure control: Circumventricular organs*

Brain stem
The pons, mid-brain and medulla oblongata.

Brattleboro rats
Strain of rat with congenital absence of antidiuretic hormone.

Breast cancer
see *Reserpine*

Bretylium tosylate
Adrenergic neurone blocking agent similar in action to guanethidine but with poor and unpredictable absorption after oral administration.
Bretylium tosylate is almost never used

Bretylium tosylate

as an antihypertensive agent now, but is
found to be a useful antiarrhythmic agent
when given parenterally for ventricular
arrhythmias resistant to other treatment.

Bromocriptine

A dopamine agonist used in the treatment
of hyperprolactinaemia and acromegaly.
In the latter disease, bromocriptine will
suppress growth hormone levels in only
50% of patients. Also the drug fails to
reduce the size of the pituitary adenoma in
acromegaly; indeed growth of the tumour
during treatment has been reported. Thus,
surgery is the treatment of choice in most
acromegalics followed by postoperative
bromocriptine if growth hormone excess
persists. See also *Acromegaly: Dopamine*

Bronchogenic carcinoma

A malignant tumour of the lung.
One histological type, oat cell carcinoma,
is a frequent source of ectopic ACTH
production and very rarely, therefore,
may cause hypertension. See also *ACTH:
Cushing's syndrome*

Bruit

Loud murmur heard on auscultation
indicative of turbulent blood flow.
Arterial stenosis may produce an abnormal
bruit, for example, in a renal artery
stenosis an abdominal bruit is heard, and
in carotid artery stenosis a bruit in the
neck is observed. Synonymous with
murmur.

Bumetanide

A loop diuretic with similar properties to
frusemide, but much more potent on a
weight for weight basis. Structurally
unrelated, however.

Bunolol

Non-cardioselective beta-adrenergic
blocking agent.

C

Cadmium

A metal, the salts of which are toxic. In a study by Schroeder in 1965 people dying from hypertension were found to have significantly higher concentrations of cadmium than people dying of other causes. Others have found similar associations and cadmium-induced hypertension was reported in one study of female rats. Hypertension is not a prominent feature in industrial cadmium poisoning, and the hypertensive effects of cadmium in man remain speculative.

Caffeine

A naturally-occurring methylxanthine, found in coffee and tea, that raises blood pressure in normal volunteers and hypertensive subjects who have abstained from recent caffeine ingestion. The haemodynamic responses to caffeine are reduced following chronic consumption. Pressor effect may be mediated by elevations in the activity of the sympathetic nervous system, by activation of the renin-angiotensin system, or by blockade of vasodilatory adenosine receptors. Recently advocated for treatment of orthostatic hypotension in patients with autonomic failure.

CAH

see *Congenital adrenal hyperplasia*

Calcium (special contribution from Dr D.M. Tillman, Western Infirmary, Glasgow, Scotland.)

Abnormalities of calcium metabolism associated with hypertension

Calcium plays a central role in modulating vascular smooth muscle tone, and hence peripheral resistance.

An abnormality of calcium metabolism may be important in the pathogenesis of primary (essential) hypertension. Several studies have shown a positive correlation between blood pressure and serum total calcium concentration. Although this may be partly explained by the effect of haemoconcentration and higher albumin concentration in hypertensive subjects, in one study, serum total calcium concentration remained significantly higher in untreated hypertensives, even after correction for albumin concentration. Urinary calcium excretion and parathyroid hormone levels are also elevated in primary hypertension, and, although the mechanisms remain imperfectly understood, hypertension frequently accompanies primary hyperparathyroidism and other hypercalcaemic conditions, including that produced by a calcium infusion.

Serum ionized calcium

The picture obtained with serum ionized calcium is less clear cut. McCarron reported that serum ionized calcium levels were reduced by approximately 0.1 mmol / l in most subjects with untreated primary hypertension. In subsequent reports by others, no difference in serum ionized calcium between hypertensives and matched normotensive controls has been observed.

Intracellular free calcium

Intracellular free calcium, the major determinant of vascular smooth muscle tone, has been shown to be increased in platelets from patients with primary hypertension. Moreover, the decrement in blood pressure (induced by beta-blocker, calcium antagonist, or diuretic therapy) correlated with the fall in cytosolic free calcium. Various other structural and functional abnormalities of cell membranes, and in particular their ion pumps have been identified in hypertensive subjects. These include abnormalities in sodium-potassium ATPase, sodium-potassium cotransport, sodium-lithium countertransport, calcium ATPase, and decreased membrane calcium binding. See also *Cell membranes: Cell sodium hypothesis: Ion transport systems*

Dietary calcium

In contrast to sodium, there is little

Calcium

information on the prevalence of hypertension and of calcium intake in populations from different countries and different cultural backgrounds. Within populations, however, calcium intake has been shown, in several studies, to be negatively correlated with blood pressure levels. Interpretation of the results of the largest of these studies, the United States National Health and Nutrition Examination Survey (NHANES-1) has been the subject of much debate, and some criticism. Further evidence is needed, ideally from prospective studies employing more objective methods of measuring calcium intake than 24-hour dietary recall.

Dietary modification
The blood pressure response to dietary calcium supplementation, one gram daily, in subjects with mild to moderate hypertension, has been reported. After eight weeks supplementation, no significant change in either blood pressure nor in serum ionized calcium was seen in normotensive controls. In contrast, there were modest, but significant, decrements in blood pressure in the 48 hypertensives, and serum ionized calcium was significantly increased. Longer term studies, however, are required before firm conclusions can be drawn.

Summary
Intracellular free calcium levels control vascular smooth muscle contraction and, therefore, total peripheral vascular resistance, which is increased in primary hypertension. Evidence is growing that calcium metabolism is altered in primary hypertension but whether this is a secondary or a causal relationship remains unclear. It is, however, possible that altered calcium handling by cell membranes acts as the final common pathway for a number of disparate abnormalities of cellular physiology associated with primary hypertension. A role for dietary calcium intake, as a determinant of arterial pressure remains speculative. It is certainly premature to advocate an increase in dietary calcium as a means of controlling hypertension in the general population.

Calcium as an intracellular second messenger
In some cells, increased cytoplasmic calcium concentration can be triggered by membrane depolarization (*voltage-dependent calcium mobilization*). A wide variety of hormones, neurotransmitters and other substances also produce their effects by increasing the concentration of calcium in the cytoplasm (*agonist-dependent calcium mobilization*). Calcium enters the cytoplasm mainly either by flowing across the plasma membrane or by being released from the sarcoplasmic reticulum in cardiac and skeletal muscle or the endoplasmic reticulum in other cells. Mitochondria also contain calcium stores. The increased cytoplasmic calcium concentration may then stimulate protein kinase C either alone or in concert with diacylglycerol. Calcium can also activate other enzymes directly, for example phospholipase A_2. Finally, calcium can bind to intracellular receptor proteins including calmodulin and troponin C. The calcium-receptor complex can then regulate a wide range of cellular activities including adenylate cyclase. (Figure 24) See also *Depolarization*

Calcium antagonists

(*also known as* Calcium channel blockers: Calcium entry blockers) Calcium antagonists are drugs that lower blood pressure by relaxing vascular smooth muscle. During cellular excitation, cytoplasmic calcium is increased by entry of extracellular calcium and by release of calcium from the sarcoplasmic reticulum. Calcium antagonists appear to act primarily by reducing calcium influx across the cell membrane preventing stimulation of contraction by the calcium-calmodulin complex.

There are three main groups of calcium antagonists:

Calcium channels

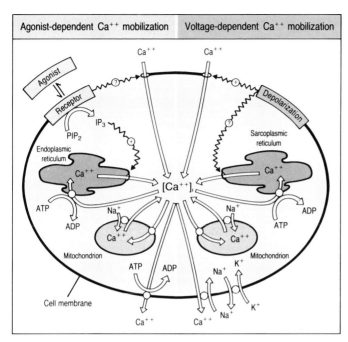

Figure 24 Calcium.
Agonist-dependent
and voltage-dependent
calcium mobilization

ADP = Adenosine
diphosphate

ATP = Adenosine
triphosphate

PIP_2 = Phosphatidyl-
inositol 4,5-bisphos-
phate

IP_3 = Inositol 1,4,5-
trisphosphate

Dihydropyridines for example,
nifedipine, nitrendipine, nimodipine,
nicardipine, felodipine.
Verapamil-like drugs for example,
verapamil, gallopamil, tiapamil.
Benzothiazepines for example, diltiazem.
The effects of representatives of each
group *in vivo* on various parameters is
indicated in Table 9. See also *Diltiazem:
Nifedipine: Verapamil*

Calcium ATPase see *Calcium pumps*

Calcium channel blockers
see *Calcium antagonists*

Calcium channels

Depolarization in some cells (including
vascular smooth muscle cells) apart
from stimulating calcium release from
intracellular stores, causes opening of
voltage-dependent calcium channels in the
plasma membrane.
These channels are the site of action of
the dihydropyridine calcium agonists and
antagonists. Agonists for these channels
stabilize the channel in the 'open' state,
and antagonists in the 'closed' state.
In agonist-dependent calcium mobilization
binding of an agonist to, for example,
an alpha₁-receptor in the cell membrane

Table 9 Calcium antagonists–A summary of the pharmacological properties *in vivo*

Parameter	Nifedipine	Verapamil	Diltiazem	
(1) Myocardial contractility	↑+	↓+	↑↓	↑=increased;
(2) Vascular muscle tone	↓++++	↓+++	↓++	↓=decreased;
(3) Heart rate	↑	↓↑	↓	↑↓=either increased or decreased;
(4) Atrioventricular conduction	0 to↑	↓++++	↓+++	o=no effect

55

Calcium channels

appears to lead to 'opening' of another, less well defined, group of calcium channels as well as stimulation of formation of inositol trisphosphate (IP_3). IP_3 then causes release of calcium from the endoplasmic reticulum (*see* Figure 24). See also *Inositol lipid metabolism*

Calcium-dependent potassium channels
Cell membrane potassium channels which open in response to a raised concentration of calcium at the internal surface of the membrane.
If, experimentally, a strong depolarizing stimulus is applied to a neuronal membrane for a long time a series of action potentials occurs with accumulation of cytoplasmic calcium. This opens the calcium-dependent potassium channels, makes the membrane harder to depolarize and increases the delay between action potentials. The calcium-dependent potassium channels are responsible for adaptation in which a continuously stimulated neurone becomes gradually less responsive.

Calcium excretion
Abnormalities of calcium excretion which have been associated with hypertension include enhanced urinary calcium excretion in the adult spontaneously hypertensive rat and a failure of the young animals to appropriately diminish calcium excretion when placed on a calcium-deficient diet. See also *Calcium*

Calcium ionophores
Proteins which facilitate the transport of calcium across cell membranes. See also *Calcium channels: Calcium pumps*

Calcium pumps
Cell membrane proteins which are necessary to transport calcium out of the cytoplasm against the concentration gradient (*see* Figure 24). Both the cell membrane and the endoplasmic and sarcoplasmic reticula have ATP-dependent

calcium pumps (ATPases). See also *Calcium-sodium exchange*

Calcium-sodium exchange
In addition to ATP-dependent calcium pumps, many excitable cells also have a sodium-calcium exchanger in the cell membrane. This is true of cardiac muscle cells and there is probably also a sodium-calcium exchange in smooth muscle cells. However, its physiological role is still contentious. See also *Blaustein hypothesis*

Callicreins see *Kallikreins: Kinins*

Calmodulin
A ubiquitous intracellular calcium receptor protein with 148 amino acid residues. Related to troponin C. Calmodulin undergoes a marked conformational change on binding calcium. The Ca^{2+}-calmodulin complex can then regulate a variety of intracellular processes and enzymes including smooth muscle contraction, secretion, microtubule disassembly, and adenylate cyclase (Figure 25). In skeletal and cardiac muscle, calcium excitation-contraction coupling is mediated by troponin C. See also *Excitation-contraction coupling: Troponin C: Vascular smooth muscle*

cAMP (Cyclic adenosine $3',5'$-monophosphate)
see *Adenosine $3',5'$-cyclic phosphate*

Canrenoate potassium
Canrenoate is a hydrolytic product of canrenone.
Conversion is catalyzed by an enzyme. Canrenoate has no intrinsic activity, but can act by its interconversion with canrenone. Potassium salt (canrenoate potassium) can be given intravenously.

Canrenone
A major metabolite of spironolactone. Canrenone is also an active aldosterone antagonist.

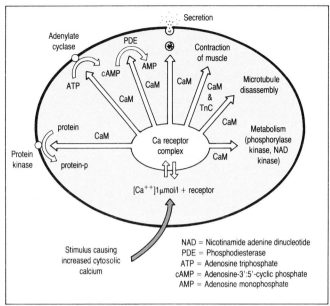

Figure 25 Calmodulin.
Calmodulin and
troponin C in the
control of many cellular
activities. Calmodulin
(CaM) is the intracellular
receptor most
commonly involved,
but troponin C (TnC) is
involved in the control
of contraction in
skeletal and cardiac
muscle

Capillary

Small blood vessels (average 8 μm
diameter) which connect the terminal
ramifications of the small arterioles with
the terminal ramifications of the small
venules.

The walls of capillaries consist of a single
layer of endothelial cells that act as
semipermeable membranes for the
interchange of various substances. They
may be continuous capillaries with an
uninterrupted endothelium as in smooth
muscle, cardiac muscle, lung; or
fenestrated capillaries when endothelial
cells have pores closed by a thin
diaphragm. These latter capillaries are
found in renal glomeruli, endocrine glands,
and in intestinal villi.

Capillary filtration

Transport of fluid with certain solutes
across the capillary endothelium. Increase
in capillary hydrostatic pressure or
decrease in capillary oncotic pressure
promotes fluid transfer to the interstitium.
See also *Starling equilibrium*

Captopril

An angiotensin I converting enzyme (ACE)
inhibitor with the structure shown
in Figure 26.

When used as sole antihypertensive agent
captopril is as effective as a thiazide or
beta-adrenergic blocking agent in lowering
blood pressure. Addition of a diuretic
controls the blood pressure of many
patients who are not controlled by
captopril alone. A steep fall in blood
pressure may occur with the initial dose,
particularly in patients with high plasma
renin concentrations, for example, those
taking diuretics or with dehydration. Renal
insufficiency may be induced in patients
with bilateral renal artery stenosis.
These properties are shared with other
converting enzyme inhibitors. Other side-
effects, such as rashes and taste loss, may
be dose-related and less common with
the lower doses now recommended.
Proteinuria may occur with pre-existing
renal disease, but does not seem to
develop in those with normal renal
function receiving total daily doses less

Captopril

than 100 mg. See also *Angiotensin I converting enzyme inhibitors: Renovascular hypertension*

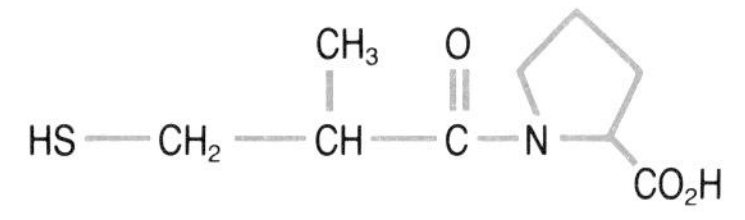

Figure 26 Captopril. Structure of captopril

Carbenoxolone

A drug, used to treat peptic ulcer, with a steroid-like structure and significant mineralocorticoid activity.
It is a semisynthetic derivative of glycyrrhizinic acid, a constituent of liquorice, and can cause hypokalaemia, fluid retention and hypertension. The clinical picture may be confused with Conn's syndrome initially, but plasma aldosterone is generally low in patients with carbenoxolone-induced hypertension. See also *Conn's syndrome: Hypokalaemia: Liquorice: Mineralocorticoid activity: Mineralocorticoid-induced hypertension*

Cardiac baroreceptors

Type A atrial stretch receptors discharge primarily during atrial systole, while type B receptors discharge mainly late in diastole.
Discharge of the latter receptors is increased when venous return is increased and they presumably respond primarily to atrial distension. The result of stimulation of these receptors is principally vasodilatation (with lowering of blood pressure) and an increase in heart rate. Experimental distension of the left ventricle produces hypotension and bradycardia, but this requires considerable distension and may not be physiologically relevant. Ventricular stretch receptors may

be involved in the maintenance of vagal tone, keeping the resting heart rate low. See also *Baroreceptors: Baroreceptors and hypertension*

Cardiac chronotropism

The ability of an agent to affect the rate of cardiac contraction.
Negative chronotropism implies that the rate is slowed, positive chronotropism that it is increased. See also *Bradycardia: Cardiac inotropism: Cardiac rate: Tachycardia*

Cardiac decompensation

Synonym for cardiac failure.

Cardiac failure (heart failure)

Failure of the heart to match its output to the metabolic needs of the body (measured as oxygen consumption) in spite of adequate filling pressures.
Left heart failure, or left ventricular failure, may occur as a consequence of severe hypertension, particularly malignant phase hypertension. Symptoms range from mild dyspnoea on exertion to florid pulmonary oedema with paroxysmal nocturnal dyspnoea and orthopnoea. Some antihypertensive drugs, especially beta-adrenergic receptor blockers, may worsen heart failure, whereas other agents, particularly angiotensin I converting enzyme inhibitors and diuretics, should be beneficial. See also *Cardiac hypertrophy*

Cardiac hypertrophy (special contribution from Professor W.A. Littler, University of Birmingham)

Pathophysiology
Hypertrophy of the left ventricle is the principal adaptation of the heart in response to systemic hypertension and its presence may predict a greater risk of mortality and morbidity. The presence of left ventricular hypertrophy in the electrocardiogram is associated with a four times greater risk in cardiovascular mortality compared with patients without evidence of hypertrophy but with similar

blood pressure levels. Long term blood pressure control has been associated with regression of left ventricular hypertrophy with most, but not all, antihypertensive agents.

Left ventricular hypertrophy can be detected within two or three days in experimental hypertension in animals. The cardiac muscle cells undergo hypertrophy and structural remodelling whilst there is hyperplasia of the non-muscular components of the myocardium such as collagen and fibrous tissue.

The hypertrophy is usually concentric but can be eccentric (interventricular septum) or irregular and may be confined to or most marked in the left ventricle. The hypertrophy may or may not be accompanied by dilatation of the left ventricle. The heart usually weighs over 500 grams (normal 300 gms) whilst the left ventricular wall is often 20 mm or more in thickness (normal 10 to 15 mm).

Left ventricular function in hypertension is largely determined by the degree of hypertrophy and the presence or absence of coronary artery disease. Hypertrophy affects both the systolic and diastolic function of the left ventricle. Whilst the increase in arterial pressure (afterload) increases the ventricular wall stress, this is offset or normalized in the early stages of hypertension by the increase in wall thickness leading to normal or supranormal systolic function. With

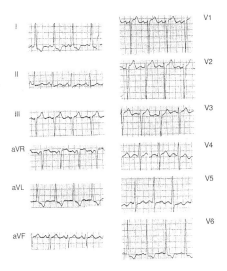

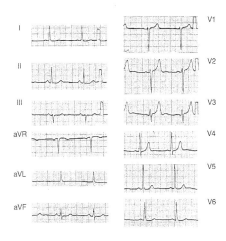

Figure 27(a) Cardiac hypertrophy. Electrocardiogram of a patient with severe hypertension showing evidence of left ventricular hypertrophy (LVH) and strain. Fulfils several criteria for LVH (See Table 10);
$S_{V1} + R_{V5} = 48$ mm;
$R_{aVL} = 15$ mm;
$R_{I} + S_{III} = 35$ mm.
Left ventricular strain pattern can be seen in leads V6, I and aVL

Figure 27(b) Cardiac hypertrophy. Electrocardiogram of the same patient as in (a) after 10 months of good blood pressure control showing disappearance of the left ventricular strain pattern. ECG changes of LVH have almost disappeared
$S_{V1} + R_{V5} = 38$ mm;
$R_{aVL} = 8$ mm;
$R_{I} + S_{III} = 20$ mm.
This probably represents regression of LVH, although echocardiography would provide better evidence of this

Cardiac hypertrophy

increasing arterial pressure and progressive ventricular dilatation there is a pathological decrease in the mass to volume ratio and an increase in peak systolic wall stress leading to depressed systolic function and ultimately left ventricular failure.
The diastolic properties of the left ventricle are adversely affected by hypertrophy leading to reduced distensibility during both the phase of passive filling of the ventricle and that of atrial contraction. Studies of the coronary circulation in hypertensive left ventricular hypertrophy are not always consistent but suggest:
The resting left ventricular blood flow in hypertensives is not different from normotensives. The maximum amount of blood flow that can be supplied to the heart is normal (coronary flow reserve) but the ability of the coronary vessels to dilate is impaired (coronary resistance). There is no simple linear relationship in hypertensive patients between the degree of left ventricular hypertrophy and the clinic recorded blood pressure. Better

correlations are achieved if ambulatory 24-hour blood pressure recordings are obtained. It is probable that the development of hypertrophy is modified by genetic, hormonal and metabolic factors, particularly adrenergic influences.
Clinical implications
Cardiac hypertrophy may be recognized during the physical examination or from the chest radiograph. The electrocardiogram and the echocardiogram are commonly used to define left ventricular hypertrophy more accurately.
Electrocardiogram (ECG)
(Figure 27 a and b)
There is a correlation between the thickness of cardiac muscle and the corresponding depolarization wave (R-wave). Hypertrophy of muscle may lead to alteration in both depolarization and repolarization with corresponding QRS-, ST- and T-wave abnormalities.
The ECG criteria for left ventricular hypertrophy are set out in Table 10.
There is evidence to suggest that currently

Figure 27(c) Cardiac hypertrophy. Echocardiograms : normal (left), patient with left ventricular hypertrophy (right). Note the increased wall thickness of the left ventricle and diminished cavity size.
RV = right ventricular cavity
IVS = interventricular septum
LV = left ventricular cavity
PVW = posterior ventricular wall

Table 10 Electrocardiographic criteria for left ventricular hypertrophy (LVH)

ECG Criterion	Sensit (%)	Specif (%)
$S_{V1} + R_{V5}$ or $R_{V6} > 35mm$	48	4
S_{V1} or $S_{V2} + R_{V5}$ or $R_{V6} > 35mm$	52	12
$S_{max\ V1\ 6} + R_{max\ V1\ 6} > 35mm$	55	16
$R_{V5} > 26mm$	28	1
$T_{V1} > T_{V6}$	69	8
$R_{aVL} > 11mm$	20	0
$R_{1}.S_{111} > 25mm$	18	0.
QRS axis > -30	18	10

Sensit = Sensitivity : those people with LVH actually identified.

Specif = Specificity : those people with normal ventricles falsely identified as having LVH
S, R, T, refer to the size of the S- wave, R - wave and T-wave respectively in the electrocardiogram.
Subscripts, for example V1, refer to the lead concerned. $S_{max\ V1-6}$ refers to the deepest
S - wave from leads V1-V6.

used ECG criteria are both insensitive and non-specific, particularly if only precordial lead criteria are used, and in young, thin-chested individuals.

Echocardiogram

Both M-mode and 2D-echocardiography are used as a non-invasive measure of left ventricular function and size in human hypertensives. Echocardiography is much more sensitive than electro-cardiography. Standard echo project-ions measure cavity dimensions and wall thickness and combinations thereof (Figure 27c). Formulae derived from these measurements give an assessment of left ventricular performance and left ventricular mass. The latter correlate well with post-mortem studies (normal LV mass 100-225 gms). However, there are problems with echocardio-graphic assessment which include image resolution, formulae used for the derivation of volume data, and 'normalizing' for body surface area. See also *Haemodynamics of systemic hypertension*

Cardiac index

The cardiac output in litres per minute divided by the body surface area in square metres. Average value is around $3\,l/min/m^2$. See also *Body surface area nomogram: Cardiac output*

Cardiac inotropism

The ability of an agent to affect the strength of cardiac contraction. Positive inotropism implies the ability of a drug, such as digoxin, to increase the force of contraction. Negative inotropism implies that the agent concerned decreases the force of contraction. Of the drugs used in the treatment of hypertension, beta-adrenergic antagonists have the most marked negative inotropic effect, and they are usually contra-indicated in the presence of cardiac failure. Occasionally they are used when it can be established that heart failure is a direct consequence of hypertension and

other agents are ineffective in lowering the blood pressure.

Of the currently available calcium antagonists, verapamil has the greatest negative inotropic effect *in vivo*. In isolated tissues, nifedipine has a greater effect, but marked vasodilatation causes reflex cardiac stimulation which over-comes the direct negative inotropic effect more than is the case with verapamil. The combined use of verapamil and a beta-adrenergic blocker orally may be particularly hazardous if myocardial function is impaired.

Cardiac output (CO)

Volume of blood pumped out of either ventricle of the heart per unit of time. Product of the stroke volume (average 0.08) and the heart rate (average 69 per minute) giving an average cardiac output (CO) of $5.5\,l/min$.

Usually measured in humans by the Fick principle, by thermodilution, or by indicator dilution (using, for example, indocyanine green or a radioactive isotope). In young subjects with mild essential hypertension CO is higher than in matched normotensive subjects. In severe hypertension CO is reduced. See also *Cardiac index: Cardiac rate: Haemodynamics of systemic hypertension: Peripheral resistance: Stroke volume*

Cardiac rate (heart rate)

Number of contractions of the ventricles of the heart per minute.

Rate of more than 100 per minute is termed tachycardia. Rate of less than 60 per minute is termed bradycardia. Heart rate is regulated by the heart's para-sympathetic and sympathetic nervous supplies. In general stimuli which increase heart rate also increase blood pressure, for instance, exercise, anger, and stimuli which cause slowing of cardiac rate usually also cause lowering of blood pressure. Important exceptions are stimulation of atrial stretch receptors in

Cardiac rate (heart rate)

which increased heart rate generally accompanies lowering of blood pressure, and the Cushing's reflex where increased intracranial pressure causes arterial hypertension accompanied by brady-cardia. Increased resting heart rate is a weak predictor of the future development of hypertension. It is often wrongly assumed that patients who have high heart rates and high blood pressures in the clinic or surgery have normal blood pressures elsewhere. Young subjects with mild essential hypertension have higher resting heart rates than normotensive controls. See also *Autonomic function tests: Cardiac output: Haemodynamics of systemic hypertension*

Cardioaccelerator

This word means causing an increase in heart rate, or it can mean an agent causing an increase in heart rate.
See also *Cardiac rate*

Cardioactive

Affecting the action of the heart. See also *Cardiac chronotropism: Cardiac inotropism*

Cardioangiography

see *Angiocardiography*

Cardiocyte

A heart muscle cell.

Cardiodynamics

The study of the motions and forces involved in cardiac contraction. See also *Haemodynamics of systemic hypertension*

Cardiogenic hypertension

Increased blood pressure with increased peripheral resistance caused by pressor reflexes originating from the heart, coronary arteries or aorta.
Hypertension thought to be related to cardiogenic pressor reflexes is paroxysmal, for example, hypertension

associated with stress, angina, myocardial infarction and dissecting aortic aneurysm.

Cardiogenic pressor reflexes

Reflexes originating from the heart and great vessels.
The heart has a sympathetic input via its afferent sympathetic nerve fibres and a parasympathetic input via the vagus nerve. Excitation of these two inputs produces complex haemodynamic effects including hypertension or hypotension. See also *Cardiogenic hypertension*

Cardiogram

A record of a cardiac event made by a cardiograph. See also *Ballistocardiogram: Echocardiogram: Electrocardiogram*

Cardiograph

An instrument which records graphically some aspect of cardiac function.

Cardiography

Technique for recording graphically aspects of cardiac function.

Cardioinhibitory centre

Area in the medulla that produces the tonic vagal discharge at rest.
It is formed by the nucleus ambiguus and related areas and receives afferents from the baroreceptors. Impulses generated by the baroreceptors (in response to increased blood pressure) excite the cardioinhibitory centre causing increased vagal tone with slowing of the heart rate. See also *Baroreceptors: Medulla oblongata*

Cardiokinetic

This word means stimulating cardiac contraction, or it can mean an agent which stimulates the contraction of the heart. See also *Cardiac chronotropism: Cardiac inotropism*

Cardiology

The branch of medicine concerned with

the heart and its function, physiological and pathological.

Cardiomyopathy
Disorder of the heart muscle of unknown cause or association.
In congestive (dilated) cardiomyopathy there is cardiac dilatation with poor systolic contraction and high end diastolic volume.
In hypertrophic cardiomyopathy there is impaired diastolic filling which may be accompanied by outflow obstruction caused by idiopathic hypertrophy of the ventricular muscle. Hypertrophic cardiomyopathy is often inherited as an autosomal dominant with incomplete penetrance.
Restrictive cardiomyopathy is characterized by impaired diastolic filling and may be caused by endomyocardial fibrotic lesions or occasionally myocardial infiltration.

Cardiopathy
Any disease of the heart. For example, hypertensive cardiopathy is heart disease caused by high blood pressure. See also *Cardiac failure: Cardiac hypertrophy: Ischaemic heart disease*

Cardiopulmonary
Pertaining to the heart and lungs. See also *Cardiopulmonary receptors: Cardiopulmonary volume*

Cardiopulmonary receptors
There is evidence for the existence of low pressure vagally innervated stretch receptors in the cardiopulmonary region. Activation of these receptors by blood volume expansion leads to decreased sympathetic input to the juxtaglomerular cells with decreased renin release. Inhibition of these receptors, for example, caused by haemorrhage, or interruption of their vagal afferent fibres, leads to increased renin release as a result of increased discharge in the renal sympathetic nerves. In this way detection of small changes in blood volume by the cardiopulmonary receptors may stimulate compensatory changes in plasma renin concentration. See also *Baroreceptors: Renin: Sympathetic nervous system*

Cardiopulmonary volume (CPV)
Blood volume contained within the heart and lungs.
Values for essential hypertensive patients tend to be lower than normal. The ratio CPV/TBV (total blood volume) is a measure of central redistribution of blood volume. It tends to be increased in patients with essential hypertension.

Cardioselectivity
Beta-adrenergic receptor blocking drugs are said to be cardioselective if they are relatively specific antagonists for the $beta_1$-receptor.

Cardiotonic
This word means having a tonic effect on the myocardium, or it can mean an agent with a tonic effect on the heart muscle. See also *Cardiac inotropism: Tone*

Cardiovascular homeostasis
The ability of control systems within the cardiovascular system to adjust the internal environment in response to changes in the external environment.

Cardiovascular system
System consisting of the heart and blood vessels.

Carotid arteries
The carotid arteries are the main vessels supplying blood to the head and neck. The left common carotid artery arises from the aortic arch in front and to the right of the origin of the left subclavian artery. The right common carotid artery begins behind the right sternoclavicular joint at the bifurcation of the innominate artery. The common carotid arteries divide at the level of C4 into the external and internal carotid arteries. The external carotid arteries end

Carotid arteries

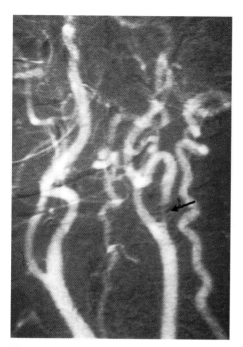

Figure 28 Carotid artery disease. Digital subtraction arteriogram showing an internal carotid artery stenosis (arrowed)

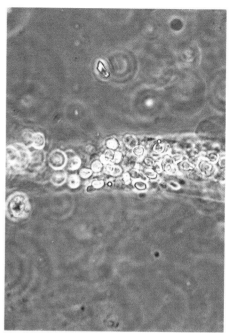

Figure 29 Casts. A red cell cast

within the parotid gland at the level of the mandible by dividing into the superficial, temporal and internal maxillary arteries. The internal carotid arteries are each dilated at their origin forming the carotid sinus where the carotid baroreceptors are found. At the base of the skull they each enter the carotid canal, then pass through the cavernous sinus and end by dividing into the anterior and middle cerebral arteries.

Carotid artery disease
Usually applies to atherosclerosis affecting the carotid arteries and their major branches (Figure 28).
More common in hypertensive patients and very common in those with transient ischaemic attacks and those who sustain a cerebral infarction. In one series of 306 consecutive patients with strokes

50% of those with carotid artery disease had previously received treatment for hypertension and a further 12% were hypertensive on admission to hospital.

Carotid receptors
see *Arterial baroreceptors: Baroreceptors*

Carotid sinus syncope
Pressure on the carotid sinus, for example from a tight collar, may cause fainting due to marked bradycardia and vasodilatation as a result of baroreceptor stimulation. See also *Cardioinhibitory centre: Carotid arteries*

Carteolol
A beta-adrenergic antagonist. See also *Beta-adrenergic receptor blocking drugs*

Casts
Cylindrical proteinaceous debris found in the urine, some of which, particularly red cell casts, imply glomerular disease (Figure 29).
A few hyaline casts may be present in normal urine, but granular casts imply underlying renal disease. Casts increase with exercise in normal subjects. Examination of the urine for casts is essential if there is significant proteinuria. See also *Chronic renal failure: Haematuria*

CAT scan
see *Computed tomography*

Catechol
1,2-benzene-diol (Figure 30).
The compound which represents the aromatic moiety of catecholamine structures, but is not an intermediate in either catecholamine synthesis or degradation. See also *Adrenaline: Catecholamines*

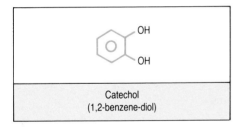

OH

OH

Catechol
(1,2-benzene-diol)

Figure 30 Catechol. Structure of catechol

Catechol-O-methyltransferase (COMT)
An important enzyme catalyzing the initial steps in catecholamine degradation. COMT, particularly in the liver, has a major role in metabolizing endogenous circulating and administered catecholamines. It is found throughout the body including the brain. Intracellular location is largely in the cytoplasm. See also *Catecholamine metabolites: Monoamine oxidase*

Catecholamine-containing neurones
Nerve cells which contain adrenaline, noradrenaline or dopamine and use one of them as a neurotransmitter. See also *Adrenaline: Central catecholamines: Dopamine: Noradrenaline: Sympathetic nervous system*

Catecholamine metabolites
The compounds produced when catecholamines are degraded (Figure 31). Measurement of some of them, particularly vanillylmandelic acid (VMA,3-methoxy 4-hydroxymandelic acid) and in some cases, normetadrenaline (NMA) in urine, is often used as a screening test for phaeochromocytoma. Confirmation, however, requires measurement of plasma catecholamines and imaging techniques. See also *Catechol-O-methyltransferase: Monoamine oxidase*

Catecholaminergic
Stimulated by or secreting one of the catecholamines. See also *Catecholamines*

Catecholamines
The group of compounds which includes adrenaline, noradrenaline and dopamine. See also *Adrenaline: Catecholamine metabolites: Catecholamines and hypertension: Central catecholamines: Dopamine: Noradrenaline*

Catecholamines and hypertension
(special contribution from Professor W.J. Louis and Dr L.G. Howes, University of Melbourne, Australia)
The concept that catecholamines may play an important role in the pathogenesis of hypertension developed progressively during the 20th century with advances in the understanding of the physiology and pharmacology of the sympathetic nervous system.
The key role the sympathetic nervous system plays in blood pressure regulation and the observation that patients with adrenal medullary tumours, (which secrete excessive amounts of

Catecholamines and hypertension

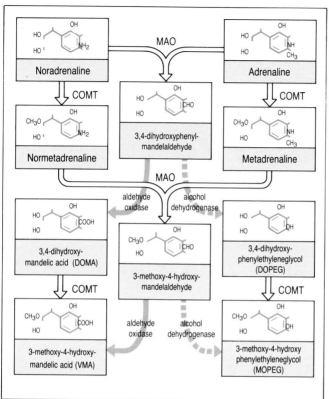

Figure 31 Catecholamine metabolites.
COMT = Catechol-O-methyltransferase;
MAO = Monoamine oxidase
VMA = Vanillylmandelic acid

catecholamines), frequently have severe hypertension, supported an association between catecholamines and elevated blood pressure.

Drugs which reduce sympathetic activity or block the action of catecholamines are used regularly in treating hypertension, and changes in both arterial and venous haemodynamics in hypertensive patients are similar to those that accompany increases in sympathetic activity.

It has, however, been difficult to obtain conclusive evidence that increased sympathetic activity is directly responsible for either the development or maintenance of most forms of clinical hypertension. This may be due, partly to a lack of sufficiently sensitive techniques for measurement of sympathetic activity in key regions, such as the central nervous system, heart, kidney and resistance blood vessels, and partly to problems with selecting control subjects in a disease where there is no clear separation between normal and high blood pressures.

Plasma noradrenaline

In the early 1970's, it was observed that plasma noradrenaline levels (which are an index of sympathetic activity) were elevated in hypertensives compared with normotensive controls. However, the recognition that factors such as age and familiarity with investigation procedures influenced plasma noradrenaline levels led to a re-evaluation of this finding. Subsequently numerous studies comparing plasma noradrenaline in hypertensives with normotensive controls

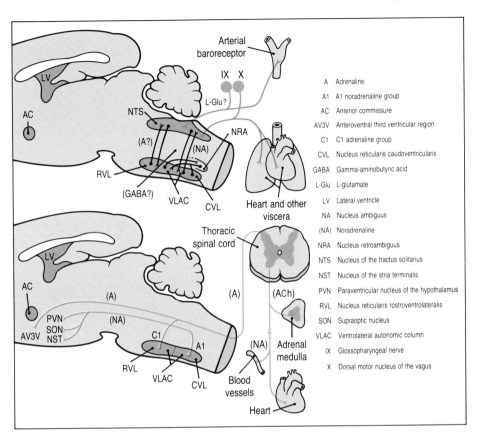

A	Adrenaline
A1	A1 noradrenaline group
AC	Anterior commissure
AV3V	Anteroventral third ventricular region
C1	C1 adrenaline group
CVL	Nucleus reticularis caudoventricularis
GABA	Gamma-aminobutyric acid
L-Glu	L-glutamate
LV	Lateral ventricle
NA	Nucleus ambiguus
(NA)	Noradrenaline
NRA	Nucleus retroambiguus
NTS	Nucleus of the tractus solitarius
NST	Nucleus of the stria terminalis
PVN	Paraventricular nucleus of the hypothalamus
RVL	Nucleus reticularis rostroventrolateralis
SON	Supraoptic nucleus
VLAC	Ventrolateral autonomic column
IX	Glossopharyngeal nerve
X	Dorsal motor nucleus of the vagus

Figure 32 Catecholamines and hypertension.
Sympathetic control of blood pressure. The upper half of Figure 32 shows the afferent inputs from the arterial baroreceptors and other viscera (possibly containing the excitatory amino acid glutamate) that terminate the nucleus of the tractus solitarius (NTS) and are important in blood pressure regulation. The lower half of Figure 32 outlines how neurones in the NTS (probably containing the inhibitory amino acid GABA) project to the rostroventrolateral medulla (RVL) which contains the C1 adrenaline-containing neurones. The C1 cells innervate the preganglionic sympathetic neurones in the intermediolateral column of the thoracic spinal cord and the AV3V region of the forebrain. Stimulation of the C1 cells leads to a pressor response due to increased sympathetic nerve discharge in the heart, blood vessels and adrenal medulla. The NTS also projects to the caudal ventrolateral medulla (CVL) which contains Al noradrenaline neurones innervating the hypothalamus. In addition the NTS projects to the vagal complex controlling the parasympathetic outflow (the cardioinhibitory centre). Supramedullary input to the NTS is also important in controlling the cardio-vascular system. Such brain regions include the cortex, amygdaloid complex and hypo-thalamus. In addition to this central control of blood pressure, catecholamines in the heart and blood vessels and catecholamines secreted from the adrenal medulla, contribute to blood pressure regulation

Catecholamines and hypertension

were published, many of which were of low statistical power and therefore inconclusive. However, when evaluated as a group, these studies suggest a small increase in plasma noradrenaline levels in hypertensives.

It is not surprising that differences in plasma noradrenaline between hypertensives and normotensives are small and inconsistent, because the contribution of organs which are important for cardiovascular regulation to total plasma noradrenaline levels is relatively small. Furthermore, plasma noradrenaline levels are not only dependent upon the rate at which noradrenaline is released from sympathetic nerves, but also the rate at which noradrenaline is cleared from plasma. This realization led to the development of techniques which selectively measure noradrenaline release from individual organs. Studies using these techniques have provided evidence for increased sympathetic activity in the heart and kidney of hypertensives, particularly in those below 40 years of age and has led to the hypothesis that increased sympathetic activity is important early in the development of hypertension, but as the disease progresses subsequent progressive vascular and cardiac hypertrophy become the major contributors to the elevated blood pressure.

Brain catecholamine pathways
Extensive studies in animal models of brain catecholamine pathways which are involved in blood pressure regulation have identified potential roles for the nucleus of the tractus solitarius and the adrenaline-containing neurones of the C1 region of the ventrolateral medulla (the vasomotor centre) in the development of hypertension. Activity in these regions is modified by supramedullary and baroreceptor pathways.

Adrenaline
The role that adrenaline plays in the pathogenesis of human hypertension is uncertain. Adrenaline released from the adrenals is capable of increasing noradrenaline release from sympathetic nerves by stimulating presynaptic beta receptors. Persistent modest elevations of plasma adrenaline have been shown to produce sustained hypertension in animal models via this mechanism. However, evidence for increased adrenaline secretion in human hypertension is lacking. (Figure 32)

Cathepsin D
A widely distributed aspartyl protease related to renin.

Cathepsin D can catalyze hydrolysis of angiotensinogen to form angiotensin I at pH below 6.0. Cathepsin D is not very active against angiotensinogen under normal circumstances, but is very active against other peptide substrates. See also *Aspartyl proteases: Renin*

CBG
see *Cortisol binding globulin*

CCK-PZ
see *Cholecystokinin-pancreozymin*

Cell membranes
Disturbances in several membrane ion transport processes have been found in essential hypertension. Altered composition of the lipid portion of the cell membrane may be a common underlying factor. Functions such as phosphoinositol turnover, calcium binding, and calcium efflux are influenced by the lipid composition, and the latter may be the link between membrane disturbances, intracellular calcium, vascular smooth muscle contraction and hypertension. Some groups have postulated that abnormalities in the distribution of sodium across the cell membrane leads to inhibition of vascular sodium-calcium exchange with increased intracellular calcium and increased vascular contractility. See also *Blaustein hypothesis: Calcium: Cell sodium hypothesis: Ion transport systems*

Cell sodium hypothesis

In certain well-defined clinical and experimental situations sodium retention causes high blood pressure, for example, in dialysis patients after bilateral nephrectomy. Amongst several explanations of this phenomenon (for example, the Guyton hypothesis) one of the most popular hypotheses postulates an effect of sodium retention on the resistance vessel smooth muscle.

Waterlogging theory
The most longstanding suggestion put forward by Professor Tobian of Minnesota, USA, is that sodium or water retention cause waterlogging which increases the resistance to blood flow. Increased arterial sodium has indeed been demonstrated in association with hypertension, but it is difficult to differentiate cause and effect. Thus the thickening of the arterial wall in larger blood vessels is associated with an increased content of collagen which binds sodium, and the extracellular fluid space of the arterial wall will also be enlarged. The increased arterial wall thickening in hypertension is associated with increased contractility and it is difficult to see how waterlogging could produce this effect. For these reasons this hypothesis is now not generally held.

Global disturbance theory
A more popular hypothesis now postulates an abnormality in transmembrane sodium fluxes which affects both vascular smooth muscle and other body cells. Evidence for this hypothesis is based partly on studies of circulating blood cells. Several studies have reported increased sodium-lithium countertransport across the red cell membrane and decreased sodium pump activity in the leucocyte. In some studies sodium-potassium cotransport has been decreased and in other studies increased.

Circulating inhibitor theories
One popular hypothesis attributes hypertension to an inhibition of sodium-calcium exchange as a result of impaired sodium pump activity due to release of a digoxin-like sodium transport inhibitor.

Intrinsic abnormality theories
Other groups have suggested that there is a global disturbance of cell membrane function for which these transport processes act as a marker. In this case changes in cell sodium are not an essential prerequisite to the development of hypertension. It is notable in this context that transport processes such as sodium-lithium countertransport probably reflect a process *in vivo* which exchanges one internal sodium for one external sodium and so would not be expected to influence cell sodium.

Relationship with cell calcium
The association between the cell membrane abnormality and blood pressure is uncertain, but amongst the possibilities put forward are changes in cellular handling of calcium causing an increase in free intracellular calcium and hence smooth muscle contractility. Alternatively slight depolarisation of vascular smooth muscle would open calcium channels and increase smooth muscle contraction.
A further hypothesis is that the abnormality of cell membrane function exerts its effect presynaptically, that is at the sympathetic nervous system level rather than the level of vascular smooth muscle. See also *Blaustein hypothesis: Cell membranes: Guyton hypothesis: Intracellular cations in essential hypertension: Ion transport systems*

Central catecholamines

The brain has three separate neuronal systems using dopamine, noradrenaline and adrenaline respectively as neuro-transmitters.
Dopaminergic neurones include ultrashort neurones in the retina and periglomerular cells of the olfactory bulb; intermediate-length neurones in the hypothalamus; and long projections between nuclei in the substantia nigra and ventral tegmentum and their targets in the striatum, in the limbic zones of the cortex and in other major regions of the limbic system.

Central catecholamines

Noradrenergic neurones arise either in the locus ceruleus of the pons or are found in the lateral tegmental portion of the reticular formation. Neurones containing adrenaline are found in the medullary reticular formation. See also *Catecholamines: Central neurotransmitters*

Central nervous system

The brain and spinal cord. See also *Autonomic nervous system: Central nervous system and hypertension; Parasympathetic nervous system; Sympathetic nervous system*

Central nervous system and

hypertension (special contribution from Professor Alberto Zanchetti, Centro di Fisiologia Clinica e Ipertensione, Ospedale Maggiore, Milano, Italy.)
Neural mechanisms, at central, reflex and peripheral levels, can be involved in hypertension both as causative and maintaining factors. Evidence that hypertension can be initiated by neural mechanisms is mostly limited to experimental hypertension, whereas evidence for neural mechanisms maintaining elevated blood pressure is available both from animal models and observations in patients.
Possible mechanisms
Although there is a limited understanding of the relationship between genetic predisposition to hypertension and environmental stimuli capable of eliciting hypertension, neural activity can be related to development of hypertension through the mechanisms of excessive environmental stimulation, specific hypertension-inducing behavioural responses to normal environmental stimuli, and exaggerated cardiovascular responses to normal environmental stimuli.
Support for the first mechanism comes from the possibility of inducing hypertension through intense and prolonged operant conditioning in monkeys. The second possibility is illustrated by the observation of hypertension in dominant males in mice colonies, while submissive males remain normotensive. Excessive cardiovascular responses to environmental stimuli have been described in the Okamoto strain of spontaneously hypertensive rat (SHR), whose blood pressure and heart rate increase in response to stressful stimuli are much greater than those of normotensive rats. In the SHR cardiovascular hyperresponsiveness to stress is not exclusively due to hyper-responsiveness of blood vessels and the heart, as it has been shown that electrical activity in renal sympathetic nerves increases to a much greater extent in hypertensive than in normotensive rats when exposed to stressful stimuli.
An additional mechanism relating neural activity and hypertension consists of alterations in cardiovascular reflexes. The current opinion is that carotid sinus and aortic baroreflexes are readjusted in hypertension. However, this resetting does not initiate hypertension, but is secondary to the rise in blood pressure. Indeed, the same type of resetting has been found in essential and renovascular hypertension in man.
Finally, there are several lines of evidence suggesting that various interactions between neural and non-neural factors effect cardiovascular control. In particular, interactions between sympathetic activity, the renin-angiotensin system and renal sodium excretion, may play a fundamental role in hypertension.
All these interactions have the characteristics of a positive feedback system, that is of a mechanism able to cause and to maintain a rise in blood pressure. (Figure 33)
Roles of the sympathetic nervous system
The sympathetic nervous system is not only capable of directly inducing systemic vasoconstriction and hypertension, but can also release renin from the juxtaglomerular cells and hence increase

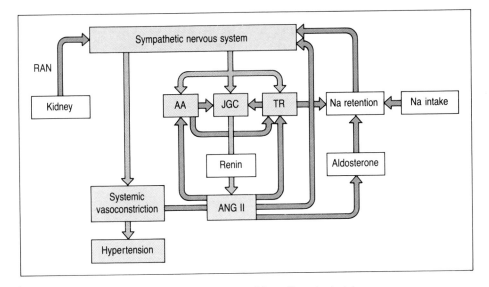

Figure 33 Central nervous system.
Positive feedback interactions between the
sympathetic nervous system and the kidney.

AA = afferent arteriole;
AngII = Angiotensin II;
JGC = juxtaglomerular cell;
RAN = renal afferent nerves;
TR = tubular reabsorption

generation of the vasoconstrictor peptide
angiotensin II. As angiotensin II is also
known to stimulate the sympathetic
nervous system both at central and
peripheral levels, the sympathetic system,
through its renin-releasing action, can also
reinforce its own activity.

Furthermore, sympathetic activity can
induce sodium retention through various
mechanisms, including a direct effect on
proximal tubular reabsorption. In turn,
sodium retention can increase sympathetic
activity, at least in hypertension-prone
subjects. Finally, these positive feedback
mechanisms might become predominant
in cardiovascular control because of a
primary or secondary weakness of
negative feedback mechanisms, such as
the sino-aortic baroreflexes. See also
*Baroreceptors and hypertension: Stress
and hypertension*

**Central neurogenic mechanisms of
experimental hypertension**
The mechanisms by which alterations in
the central nervous system cause
hypertension have been studied by
various techniques, for example, electrical
stimulation or thermocoagulative ablation
of parts of the central nervous system,
as well as use of neurotoxins. The
hypothalamus, particularly, has been
studied using electrical stimulation.
Centrally-acting antihypertensive drugs
have provided insights particularly into
the role of central catecholaminergic
systems. See also *Central nervous system
and hypertension: Centrally acting antihypertensive drugs*

Central neurotransmitters
These are substances acting as
neurotransmitters within the central
nervous system. Amino acids involved
include gamma-aminobutyrate (GABA),

Central neurotransmitters

glycine, and possibly glutamate and aspartate. Other substances include catecholamines, acetylcholine, 5-hydroxytryptamine (serotonin), and possibly histamine. Various peptides, including endorphins, atrial natriuretic peptides and so-called 'gut peptides', for instance, vasoactive intestinal polypeptide (VIP), are also thought to act as central neurotransmitters. See also *Brain peptides and blood pressure control*

Centrally acting antihypertensive drugs

Drugs such as clonidine, methyldopa and reserpine are thought to lower blood pressure primarily by interruption of central neurotransmission. For the mechanism of action of clonidine see *Alpha$_2$-agonist drugs*. Methyldopa may function by virtue of its conversion to alpha-methylnoradrenaline which acts as a false transmitter and thereby decreases sympathetic outflow from the central nervous system. Reserpine acts by depleting stores of catecholamines and 5-hydroxytryptamine in the brain and other organs. See also *Alpha-methyldopa: Clonidine: Reserpine*

Cerebellar haemorrhage

This haemorrhage into the cerebellum is more common in hypertensive patients. It presents with sudden occipital headache, vertigo, diplopia and ataxia and usually develops over, perhaps, six hours. Cerebellar haemorrhage may be accompanied by sixth cranial nerve palsy, facial weakness, dysarthria and dysphagia. Enlargement of the haematoma in the posterior cranial fossa may lead to sub-acute hydrocephalus. Surgical evacuation should be considered. See also *Cerebral haemorrhage*

Cerebral arteries

The internal carotid artery ends by dividing into the anterior cerebral artery and the middle cerebral artery. The former supplies the medial and superolateral aspects of the cerebral hemispheres, while the latter supplies the internal capsule and most of the lateral aspects of the cerebral cortex. The two anterior cerebral arteries are connected by the anterior communicating artery. The posterior cerebral arteries arise from the basilar artery and are joined to the corresponding internal carotid artery by the posterior communicating artery, completing the Circle of Willis. See also *Berry aneurysms: Cerebrovascular accident*

Cerebral circulation

Circulation of blood to the brain. It is subject to prominent autoregulation in hypertensive and normotensive patients to maintain relatively constant flow despite variations in perfusion pressure. Autoregulation may depend on an inherent ability of vascular smooth muscle to contract when stretched or upon washing away of vasodilator metabolites when perfusion pressure and flow is increased. However, whereas in normal subjects mean arterial pressure can be reduced to 60-70 mmHg without affecting cerebral blood flow, hypertensive subjects cannot tolerate this degree of blood pressure reduction, and may develop symptoms of cerebral hypoxia. See also *Autoregulation of blood flow: Cerebral hypoxia: Cerebral infarction*

Cerebral haemorrhage

Intracerebral haemorrhage is common in hypertensive patients and usually occurs by rupture of tiny Bouchard-Charcot microaneurysms. These are uncommon in normotensive individuals. About 80% of cerebral haemorrhages are located in the cerebral hemispheres. Haemorrhage presents as a vascular stroke with sudden onset of neurological deficit, for example, hemiplegia and dysphasia. There may also be headache and/or alteration in consciousness. Diagnosis of cerebral haemorrhage has been made much easier by the advent of computed tomography.

In most cases surgical evacuation of the haematoma is not indicated and only supportive treatment is available. See also *Bouchard-Charcot microaneurysms: Cerebrovascular accident: Computed tomography*

Cerebral hypoxia

The brain consumes 20% of the total resting oxygen consumption and is extremely vulnerable to hypoxia. Structures in the brain stem are much less sensitive to hypoxia than the cortex and patients may recover from, for example, cardiac arrest with normal brain stem function but severe intellectual impairment. The basal ganglia also have a high oxygen requirement and hypoxia can cause a Parkinsonian syndrome. Cerebral hypoxia in hypertensive patients may result from lowering of blood pressure below the lower limit at which autoregulation can be maintained. Localized areas of atherosclerotic narrowing in the arterial supply to parts of the brain may make these regions vulnerable to hypoxia if the blood pressure is reduced below a critical level. See also *Cerebral infarction: Hypoxia: Ischaemia*

Cerebral infarction

Ischaemic necrosis of part of the brain, which may affect a small area or a large part of the brain.

The size of the infarct depends on the degree of atherosclerosis and the available collateral circulation. Cerebral infarction may result from thrombosis of the supplying artery or occlusion of the artery by an embolus from elsewhere, often an atherosclerotic artery. Ischaemia, however, will only occur if the collateral circulation is inadequate. Cerebral infarction is more common in hypertensive patients than in age-matched normotensive controls. Atheroma affecting the carotid arteries and their major branches is often the likely source of embolism.

Cerebral infarction can be divided into cortical infarction and capsular or lacunar infarction.

Cortical infarction

Cortical infarction results from occlusion of a major artery supplying part of a cerebral hemisphere, most commonly the middle cerebral artery. Clinically, cortical infarction often presents with sudden or gradual onset of hemiplegia accompanied by dysphasia, dyspraxia or hemianopia. Cortical infarction is the commonest form of stroke and appears on computed tomographic scanning as an area of reduced density. Only supportive treatment is available for an established cerebral infarction, therefore great emphasis must be placed on prevention by modifying risk factors such as hypertension, cigarette smoking and diabetes. Transient ischaemic attacks may be warning symptoms of an impending stroke. See also *Atherosclerosis: Carotid arteries: Cerebrovascular accident: Computed tomography: Lacunar infarction: Transient ischaemic attacks*

Cerebrovascular accident

(*also known as* Stroke) This term includes both cerebral haemorrhage and cerebral infarction. Stroke is the third commonest cause of death in the developed countries after heart disease and cancer. All forms of stroke are more common in hypertensive patients and the risk seems to be related to the degree of blood pressure elevation (Figure 34).

Virtually every trial examining the effects of lowering blood pressure in hypertensive patients has shown reduction in the risk of stroke, but with milder degrees of hypertension the number of patients who need to be treated for a given period to prevent one stroke is much larger. There is also evidence to suggest that good blood pressure control in patients who have had a cerebrovascular accident before will reduce the likelihood of recurrence. See also *Cerebral haemorrhage: Cerebral infarction: Multicentre studies of clinical outcome*

Charcot-Bouchard microaneurysms

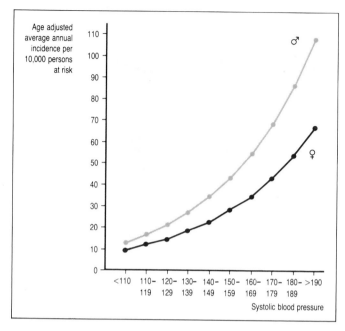

Age adjusted average annual incidence per 10,000 persons at risk

Systolic blood pressure

Figure 34 Cerebro-vascular accident. The effect of systolic blood pressure on the incidence of cerebro-vascular accident (derived from Framing-ham Study: patients aged 45–74 years with 18 years follow up)

Charcot-Bouchard microaneurysms
see *Bouchard-Charcot microaneurysms*

Chelmsford Study (Lancet 1964 1: 235-238)
The first controlled clinical trial of the treatment of uncomplicated essential hypertension. All patients had diastolic blood pressures of 110 mmHg or more. It showed clear benefit of treatment of hypertension in men although benefits were not significant in women. However, the numbers of patients were small.

Chemoreceptors
Sensory receptors which are stimulated by a change in the chemical composition of their environment. Chemoreceptors include receptors for taste and smell. See also *Circumventricular organs*

Children and hypertension
The average blood pressure in children increases with age. This is particularly true for systolic pressure which rises until the age of 20 years by an average of 2 mmHg / year in males and 1 mmHg / year in females. The 95th percentile levels for ages 3-12 years are set out in Table 11. The outcome for children whose blood pressures are consistently above given levels is unknown.
Blood pressure in children correlates with obesity and indices of body mass. Other associations include parental blood pressure, resting heart rate, and sexual maturity with acceleration of the rate of increase of blood pressure during puberty. 'Tracking' (maintenance of rank order within the distribution over time) is present in childhood, but it has a low predictive power and it is still uncertain whether individuals appearing consistently at the high end of the distribution are the hypertensives of the future.
'Horse racing' (the phenomenon where rate of increase in blood pressure in individuals is related to the absolute level at any one time) does not seem to occur in children, although there is evidence for it

in adults. The reasons for this discrepancy are not clear.

The actual level of blood pressure in childhood is the best predictor of future blood pressure level, but the predictive value of relatively high blood pressure for future hypertension is rather low. The lack of epidemiological data makes management recommendations somewhat arbitrary.

Perhaps apparently healthy children should have their blood pressure measured at least once before school and once in early adolescence. More frequent measurements seem sensible in those consistently around the 95th percentile for their age, and in those with a positive family history. Proteinuria, haematuria and very high pressures should lead to investigation for secondary hypertension. The latter becomes less common with increasing age. If treatment is thought necessary it seems reasonable to advise weight loss in the obese although the efficacy of this has not been formally proven in children. See also *Age: Elderly and hypertension*

Table 11 95th percentile blood pressure levels for ages 3-12 years	
Age (y)	95th Percentile level
3	112/78
6	116/79
9	125/82
12	135/87

Chlorisondamine chloride
A ganglion blocker now little used in the treatment of hypertension. See also *Ganglion blocking drugs*

Chlorothiazide
A thiazide diuretic used in the treatment of hypertension. See also *Thiazide diuretics*

Chlorpromazine
A major tranquillizer of the phenothiazine group of drugs, which also has complex cardiovascular side-effects.

Intravenous administration causes postural hypotension due to a combination of central actions and peripheral alpha-adrenergic blockade, and reflex tachy-cardia. Oral administration has a mild hypotensive effect (systolic more than diastolic). Tolerance usually develops to the hypotensive effect, but orthostatic hypotension may persist.

Chlorthalidone
A thiazide diuretic used in the treatment of hypertension. See also *Thiazide diuretics*

Cholecystokinin-pancreozymin (CCK-PZ)
Group of peptides containing 4-39 amino acid residues. These are found in the endocrine cells of the gut, as well as in brain and peripheral nerves. In addition to stimulating gallbladder contraction and pancreatic enzyme secretion, they have limited vasoactive properties and have been found to produce splanchnic vasodilatation and mild hypotension in anaesthetized dogs.

Cholesterol
A lipid found in cell membranes and in plasma lipoproteins.

A fasting plasma total cholesterol concentration of 6.5 mmol / l or more is associated with an appreciable risk of ischaemic heart disease. The risk seems to be directly proportional to low density lipoprotein (LDL) cholesterol level and inversely proportional to high density lipoprotein (HDL) cholesterol level.

Most people with raised plasma cholesterol concentrations have polygenic hypercholesterolaemia, which usually responds to dietary modification (optimized calorie intake, reduced saturated fats, increased ratio of poly-unsaturated to saturated fatty acids, and increased dietary fibre). Monogenic

Cholesterol

inherited causes, for example, familial hypercholesterolaemia and familial combined hyperlipidaemia, often show an inadequate response to diet alone. The choice of drug treatment depends, to some degree, on whether there is concomitant elevation of triglyceride. Drugs include cholestyramine, colestipol, probucol, bezafibrate and the new inhibitors of hydroxymethylglutaryl coenzyme A reductase (for example, mevinolin). Thyromimetic drugs (which have the cholesterol-lowering effect, but not the cardiovascular effects, of thyroxine) may also have a place in the future.

Recent studies suggest that lowering cholesterol with diet and drugs in patients with hypercholesterolaemia may reduce their incidence of and mortality from coronary artery disease, but this remains a controversial area. In addition, there is little information available on the effects of long term use of lipid lowering drugs. Cholesterol is also the precursor of the adrenocortical steroids. See also *Antihypertensive drugs and serum lipids: Familial hyperlipoproteinaemia: Secondary hyperlipoproteinaemia*

Choline

The precursor of acetylcholine, an important neurotransmitter. See also *Acetylcholine*

Table 12 Classes of cholinergic neurones and respective cholinoceptive sites

Class	Site
Postganglionic, parasympathetic	Autonomic effector cell
Preganglionic autonomic	Autonomic ganglion cell
Somatic motor	Striated muscle cell
Central nervous system cholinergic neurones	Central neurones

Choline acetyltransferase (CAT)

Enzyme which catalyzes the final step in acetylcholine synthesis. See also *Acetylcholine*

Cholinergic

Stimulated or transmitted by acetylcholine. A term also applied to neurones employing acetylcholine as a neurotransmitter. Cholinergic neurones fall into the four classes at their respective sites specified in Table 12.

Cholinergic receptors

(*also known as* Cholinoceptors) Membrane-bound proteins to which acetylcholine binds after release from a cholinergic neurone and produces a physiological response.

These receptors were originally divided into nicotinic receptors (in autonomic ganglia and on skeletal muscle end-plates) and muscarinic receptors (on autonomic effector cells). It is now known that nicotinic receptors in autonomic ganglia are different from those at skeletal muscle end plates and muscarinic receptors are also found in autonomic ganglia. Muscarinic receptors have also been subdivided into M_1 and M_2 receptors.

Cholinesterase

An enzyme which catalyzes the hydrolysis of acetylcholine. Acetylcholinesterase is responsible for the hydrolysis which occurs in the vicinity of the nerve ending after acetylcholine release. Pseudocholinesterase is present in glial cells and also in plasma. Its physiological function is unknown. See also *Acetylcholine*

Cholinoceptive sites

Term applied to sites on effector organs on which acetylcholine acts. See also *Acetylcholine: Cholinergic: Cholinergic receptors*

Cholinolytic

This word means antagonizing the action

of acetylcholine, or of cholinomimetic agents, or, it can mean a drug which blocks the effect of acetylcholine. See also *Acetylcholine: Antagonist: Cholinomimetic*

Cholinomimetic
Having a similar biological effect to acetylcholine.

Chronic bronchitis
Defined as daily cough with sputum for 3 months a year for at least 2 consecutive years.

Some degree of airways obstruction may be present in chronic bronchitis. It may be reversible to some extent. Beta-adrenergic antagonists (particularly non-cardioselective drugs) are contraindicated in asthma. They can be given to patients with chronic bronchitis and reversible airways obstruction as long as the patient is instructed to increase the use of his beta$_2$-stimulatory bronchodilator (for instance, salbutamol) if necessary. If there is any doubt, however, beta blockers should be avoided in these patients. See also *Beta-adrenergic receptor blocking drugs*

Chronic glomerulonephritis
The end result of progression of glomerulonephritis of various types. The rate of progression depends on the type of glomerulonephritis, and also varies between individuals. Reduction (usually bilateral) in renal size will be detected on an intravenous pyelogram. In over 70% of these patients there is no history to suggest preceding renal disease and it is often not possible to decide, even by histological examination, the preceding type of glomerulonephritis. Patients may present with chronic renal failure and are often hypertensive. See also *Chronic renal failure: Glomerulonephritis: Intravenous pyelography*

Chronic pyelonephritis
(*also known as* Reflux nephropathy) No

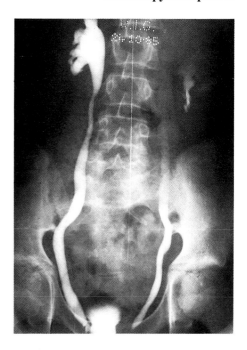

Figure 35a Chronic pyelonephritis. Micturating cystourethrogram showing bilateral vesicoureteric reflux

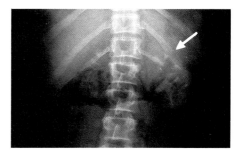

Figure 35b Chronic pyelonephritis. Intravenous pyelogram in the same patient. Note dilated calyces and polar cortical scarring in the left kidney (arrowed)

association has been reported between acute pyelonephritis and hypertension. Chronic pyelonephritis is the focal kidney scarring which develops in children under

Chronic pyelonephritis

the Age of four years with urinary tract infection and vesicoureteric reflux (Figure 35a). It is recognized on an intravenous pyelogram by cortical (usually polar) scarring and dilated calyces (Figure 35b). Chronic pyelonephritis may be associated with hypertension either in childhood or adult life, especially if scarring is severe and renal function markedly impaired. Removal of a single pyelonephritic kidney may alleviate hypertension. The mechanism of hypertension in chronic pyelonephritis is unclear (there are probably several components). See also *Chronic renal failure*

Chronic renal failure

Renal impairment in a hypertensive patient may result from prolonged severe hypertension causing nephrosclerosis or atherosclerotic renovascular disease. However, many diseases of the kidneys also cause hypertension. The presence of microscopic haematuria may, for example, indicate underlying glomerulonephritis. Casts, particularly red cell casts or casts containing red cells, imply glomerular disease. Heavy proteinuria is likely to be due to glomerulonephritis, in which case haematuria is almost invariable. The degree of renal insufficiency is usually assessed by measuring the creatinine clearance. In some patients with chronic renal failure and hypertension control of blood pressure may improve renal function or delay its deterioration. In the presence of significant renal impairment loop diuretics will be more effective antihypertensive agents than thiazides. The doses of some other agents, for example atenolol, may need to be reduced or a drug which is not excreted by the kidney substituted. See also *Chronic glomerulonephritis: Chronic pyelonephritis: Glomerulonephritis: Polycystic disease*

Chronotropism

see *Cardiac chronotropism: Cardiac inotropism*

Cigarette smoking

Blood pressure rises slightly when a cigarette is smoked, but epidemiological surveys have shown a tendency to lower readings in smokers than in non-smokers. However, cigarette smoking is a major independent risk factor for myocardial infarction, death from aortic aneurysm, peripheral vascular disease and cerebral infarction (apart from increasing the risk of non-cardiovascular diseases such as bronchial carcinoma and chronic bronchitis). Several mechanisms have been postulated to account for the relationship between smoking and atherosclerosis. Since smoking and hypertension act together in a more than additive fashion in increasing the risk of atherosclerosis, smoking should clearly be strongly discouraged in hypertensive patients. Patients who present with malignant phase hypertension have a much higher prevalence of smoking than matched patients with less severe hypertension (Figure 36). Fibromuscular dysplasia of the renal arteries is also more common in smokers. See also *Fibromuscular dysplasia: Malignant phase hypertension*

Circle of Willis

(Thomas Willis, English anatomist and physician, 1621-1675)
A polygonal anastomosis formed by some of the vessels supplying the brain. See also *Berry aneurysms: Cerebral arteries*

Circumventricular organs

Four small areas in or near the brain stem which stain like the tissues outside the brain when an acidic dye is injected intravenously into an animal. They are the posterior pituitary and the adjacent ventral part of the median eminence of the hypothalamus, the area postrema, the organum vasculosum of the lamina terminalis (OVLT), and the subfornical organ (SFO). They lie outwith the blood-brain barrier because their capillaries are fenestrated. Some circumventricular

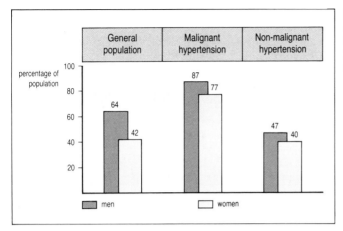

Figure 36 Cigarette smoking. Smoking is more common in patients with malignant phase hypertension

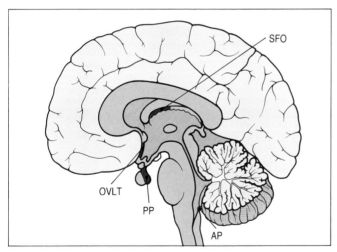

Figure 37 Circum-ventricular organs. A sagittal section of the human brain showing the OVLT and SFO (see text) as well as the posterior pituitary (PP) and the area postrema (AP)

organs act as neurohaemal organs, for example, the posterior pituitary (PP), while others act as chemoreceptor organs, for example, the area postrema. (Figure 37) See also *Blood-brain barrier: Brain renin-angiotensin system: Chemoreceptors: Neurohaemal organs*

Claudication
Pain in the muscles usually of the lower limb associated with exertion and caused by ischaemia as a consequence of atherosclerosis of the lower limb arteries (peripheral vascular disease).

More common in hypertensive patients, especially if they are smokers. See also *Atherosclerosis: Cigarette smoking: Peripheral vascular disease*

Clear cell carcinoma of kidney
(*also known as* Grawitz's tumour: Hypernephroma) A malignant tumour of the kidney. Several well-documented cases have been reported where hypertension was associated with one of these tumours and resolved with removal of the lesion. In many of these cases plasma renin activity was increased and the tumour

Clear cell carcinoma of kidney

tissue contained much more renin than the surrounding normal tissue. In some cases tumour cells have been found to contain secretory granules. See also *Renin: Renin-secreting tumours*

Clonidine

A centrally acting antihypertensive drug. It has become less popular because of the dangers associated with sudden withdrawal. A transdermal preparation has been developed. Most frequent side-effects are xerostomia and sedation. Clonidine causes fluid retention when used as sole therapy. Other side-effects include central nervous system effects, for example, insomnia, nightmares, and also skin rashes. See also *Centrally acting antihypertensive drugs*

Clonidine suppression test

A test used in the diagnosis of phaeo-chromocytoma, which is based on the principle that normal increases in plasma catecholamine concentrations are caused by activation of the sympathetic nervous system whereas in patients with phaeochromocytoma the increases result largely from diffusion of excess catecholamines from the tumour into the circulation. It is found that clonidine suppresses plasma (or urinary) catech-olamine concentrations in normal people, but not in patients with phaeochromocytoma, by decreasing sympathetic discharge. See also *Alpha₂-agonist drugs: Clonidine: Phaeo-chromocytoma*

Clonidine withdrawal syndrome

Sudden withdrawal of clonidine may cause potentially life-threatening hypertension accompanied by anxiety, headache, abdominal pain, palpitation, and sweating. It usually occurs about 20 hours after the last dose and may persist for 7-10 days. Treatment is by means of combined alpha- and beta-adrenergic blockade, or intravenous nitroprusside with intensive

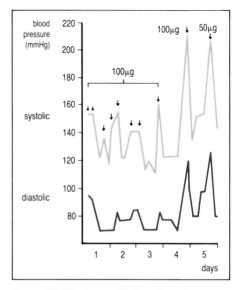

Figure 38 Clonidine withdrawal syndrome. Rebound hypertension occurring about 24 hours after the dose of clonidine on day 3

monitoring. Alternatively, clonidine can be reintroduced. (Figure 38)

Clopamide

A diuretic used in the treatment of hypertension. See also *Diuretics*

Clorexolone

A diuretic used in the treatment of hypertension. See also *Diuretics*

Coarctation of the aorta

Briefly described as the narrowing of the aortic lumen, it is a rare cause of hypertension.
In the most common variety the area of narrowing is just distal to the left subclavian artery (LSA) (Figure 39a). Occasionally the narrowing is proximal to the LSA. This congenital disorder is much commoner in males. Coarctation may be associated with a bicuspid aortic valve, with Turner's syndrome and with berry aneurysms. The characteristic clinical

finding is hypertension in the upper limbs and hypotension with a delayed femoral pulse in the lower limbs. Hypertension is usually not severe but these patients are at increased risk of cardiac failure, aortic rupture or dissecting aneurysm, infective endocarditis and subarachnoid haemorrhage (from berry aneurysms). There may be a murmur audible over the back caused by the narrowing itself or collateral circulation. A chest radiogram may show bilateral notching of the inferior margins of the ribs (Figure 39b) between the third and tenth ribs (produced by enlarged intercostal arteries). Coarctation is best demonstrated by aortography (Figure 39c). The mechanism of the hypertension is unclear. Treatment is surgical. See also *Aorta: Berry aneurysms: Cardiac failure: Dissecting aortic aneurysm: Subarachnoid haemorrhage*

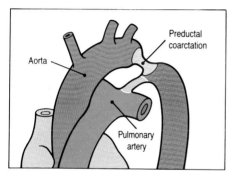

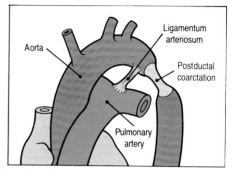

Figure 39a Coarctation of the aorta. Commonest sites of coarctation of the aorta: area of narrowing may be proximal (preductal) or distal (postductal) to the insertion of the ligamentum arteriosum

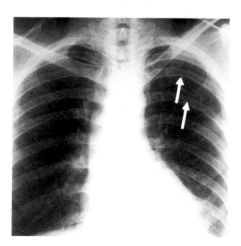

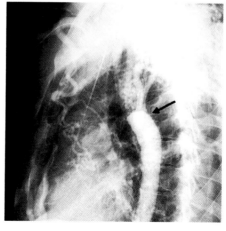

Figure 39b Coarctation of the aorta. Chest radiogram of a patient with aortic coarctation. Rib notching is marked with arrows

Figure 39c Coarctation of the aorta. Aortogram demonstrating aortic coarctation (arrowed)

Cocaine

Cocaine
In addition to its general stimulatory effects on the central nervous system, cocaine has cardiovascular effects. In moderate dosage it increases heart rate, partly by increased central sympathetic stimulation and also, by its peripheral effects on the sympathetic nervous system. (It blocks reuptake of catecholamines at adrenergic nerve endings, and potentiates neurotransmission and the effects of circulating catecholamines.) Blood pressure usually rises initially due to tachycardia and vasoconstriction, but may eventually fall.

Coffee drinking
see *Caffeine*

Cold pressor test
A test primarily of the function of the efferent sympathetic fibres of the autonomic nervous system. The hand of the subject is immersed in iced water for one minute and blood pressure is measured in the other arm at 30 seconds and one minute. In a normal subject systolic pressure will be found to rise by 16-20 mmHg and diastolic pressure should rise by 12-15 mmHg. See also *Autonomic function tests*

Collecting ducts
The distal convoluted tubules of the nephrons converge to drain into collecting ducts which are about 2 cm long and pass through the renal cortex and medulla to empty into the pelvis of the kidney at the apices of the medullary pyramids. Changes in osmolality and volume in the collecting ducts are affected by antidiuretic hormone. In the presence of antidiuretic hormone, collecting duct epithelium is more permeable to water and concentrated urine is produced. See also *Convoluted tubules: Nephron*

Compliance
Apparent failure of medication to control blood pressure is often due to the patient's failure to take all the medication prescribed (poor drug compliance). Another feature which may arouse suspicion is failure of the heart rate to slow while apparently taking a beta-adrenergic receptor blocking drug. Perhaps 50% of non-compliers will admit non-compliance. Strategies to improve compliance include, keeping the drug regime as simple as possible, advising the patient to, for example, take his medication 'with breakfast' rather than 'once a day'. Obviously, compliance is likely to be poorer if there are unpleasant side-effects of the drug. See also *Arterial compliance*

Complications of hypertension
Many hypertensive patients are not identified or treated until complications occur. The effects of hypertension on so-called 'target organs' are described in Figure 40. The presence of target organ damage at presentation may be an adverse prognostic feature. Hypertensive complications can be divided into atherosclerotic (which occur in normal individuals, but earlier or to a greater degree in hypertensive patients) or truly hypertensive. In general, the main exception being cerebral infarction, treatment has been more effective in preventing the latter group.

Computed tomography (CT)
(*also known as* Computerized tomography scans: Computerized axial tomography (CAT) scans) Radiological technique in which the emergent x-ray beam is measured by a scintillation counter, the electronic impulses are recorded digitally and processed by a computer to yield a reconstructed cross-section of part of the body. CT scanning of the brain is useful in differentiating cerebral haemorrhage from cerebral infarction. See also *Adrenal computed tomography*

Congenital adrenal hyperplasia (CAH)
Adrenal hyperplasia resulting from an

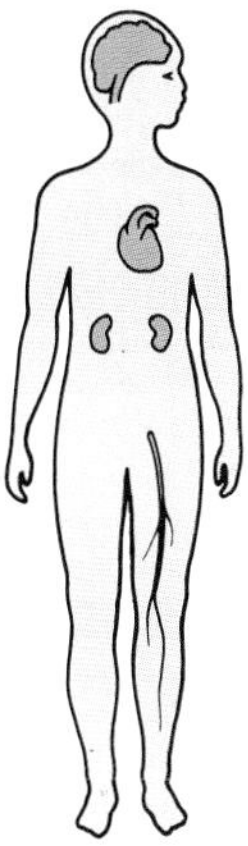

	TARGET ORGANS	ATHEROSCLEROTIC	HYPERTENSIVE
	Brain	a) transient ischaemic attacks b) cerebral infarction	a) hypertensive encephalopathy b) cerebral haemorrhage
	Eyes	retinal vascular accident eg. retinal vein occlusion	hypertensive retinopathy
	Heart	a) angina pectoris b) myocardial infarction	a) cardiac hypertrophy b) cardiac failure
	Kidneys	renal vascular disease	a) nephrosclerosis b) fibrinoid necrosis
	Peripheral arteries	a) intermittent claudication b) gangrene	a) arterial aneurysms b) aortic dissection

Figure 40 Complications of hypertension

inborn error which impairs the efficiency of any step in the biosynthesis of cortisol. Hyperplasia is stimulated by the compensatory increase in ACTH. Commonest variety is 21-hydroxylase deficiency with impaired synthesis of aldosterone as well as cortisol. Second most common is 11β-hydroxylase deficiency. See also *Hyperplasia*

Congenital mesoblastic nephroma
A tumour of the kidney which sometimes produces renin. Incidence is only about 10% that of nephroblastoma. Nephrectomy is usually curative and, where renin is secreted, has returned plasma renin activity to normal. See also *Renin-secreting tumours*

Congestive heart failure
see *Cardiac failure (heart failure)*

Conn's syndrome
(Jerome W. Conn, U.S. physician, born 1907)
Strictly speaking, this term applies to primary aldosteronism caused by an adrenocortical adenoma, but it is used by some to refer to all causes of aldosteronism with low plasma renin activity. Separation of aldosteronism with bilateral

hyperplasia, or occasionally histologically normal adrenals, from Conn's syndrome proper is justified as this 'non-tumorous aldosteronism' may actually represent a variant of essential hypertension.
  Symptoms
Patients with Conn's syndrome may present with symptoms of hypokalaemia, for example, muscle weakness, polyuria, polydipsia, paraesthesiae or tetany. They are often symptomless.
  Diagnosis
Diagnosis is suggested by low serum potassium concentrations with high to normal concentrations of sodium. Raised plasma aldosterone is accompanied by suppressed plasma renin activity (Figure 41). Localization of the adenoma is often possible by non-invasive methods, for example, CT scanning or adrenal scintigraphy, but the most reliable method is still adrenal venous sampling with measurements of plasma aldosterone.
  Treatment
Treatment is generally by surgical removal of the adrenal gland containing the adenoma after blood pressure and electrolyte disturbances have been brought under control with spironolactone or amiloride. See also *Adrenal cortex:*

83

Conn's syndrome

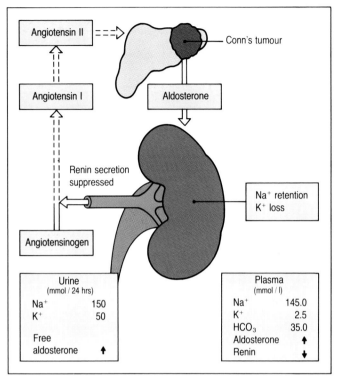

Figure 41 Conn's syndrome. Primary aldosteronism due to an aldosterone-secreting adreno-cortical adenoma: biochemical effects

Adrenal adenomas: Adrenal computed tomography: Adrenal scintigraphy: Adrenal ultrasonography: Adrenal venography: Adrenal venous sampling: Mineralocorticoid-induced hypertension

Contraceptive pill

A rise in blood pressure occurs in virtually all women who take the combined oral contraceptive for six months or more. The incidence of hypertension (blood pressure $\geqslant 140/90$ mmHg) in these women is perhaps 4-5%. There appears to be general agreement that the oestrogenic component of the combined oral contraceptive is involved in causing 'pill-induced hypertension' but whether or not the progestogen contributes is less clear. The progestogen-only oral contraceptive probably has little, if any, effect on blood pressure.

Oral contraceptive-induced hypertension may be severe and cases of malignant phase hypertension have been reported. Blood pressure should be checked prior to commencing the oral contraceptive and at regular intervals (at least six-monthly) while it is being taken. The oral contraceptive should be avoided in patients with pre-existing hypertension, diabetes mellitus, hyperlipidaemia, and those who are smokers because of the increased risk of atherosclerosis. If persistent hypertension is noted while taking the combined oral contraceptive, a change to a progestogen-only oral contraceptive or an alternative form of contraception may be all that is required. On withdrawal of the combined oral contraceptive blood pressure usually returns to normal within three months. If blood pressure is still elevated after six months an alternative explanation for the hypertension should be considered, although oral contraceptive-induced hypertension can be persistent. If blood pressure remains high, treatment with antihypertensive drugs may become necessary. If contraception is vital and no other method is acceptable it is occasionally justifiable to prescribe both the oral contraceptive pill and an antihypertensive drug, but only in exceptional circumstances.

Contractility
Capacity for shortening when an appropriate stimulus is applied.

Converting enzyme
see *Angiotensin I converting enzyme*

Converting enzyme inhibitors
see *Angiotensin I converting enzyme inhibitors*

Convoluted tubules
Segments of the nephron. The proximal convoluted tubule (PCT) is distal to Bowman's capsule. It terminates in the thin segment of the descending limb of the loop of Henle. The distal convoluted tubule (DCT) is distal to the loop of Henle. Distal convoluted tubules from a number of nephrons drain into a collecting duct. The tubules are concerned with reabsorption and secretion of various substances. See also *Bowman's space: Collecting ducts: Glomerulus: Nephron*

Coope's Study of Hypertension in the Elderly (British Medical Journal 1986, 293:1145-1151)
An open study without placebo comparing the effect of antihypertensive treatment (n=419) against no antihypertensive treatment (n=465) for a mean follow-up of 4.4 years in subjects aged 60-79 years. Antihypertensive drugs, mainly atenolol and bendrofluazide, were introduced in a stepwise manner. The study included patients with either systolic pressure

≥ 170 mmHg or diastolic pressure ≥ 105 mmHg, hence, unlike the EWPHE study, it included patients with isolated systolic hypertension. The study showed that drug treatment significantly reduced fatal strokes and total (fatal and non-fatal) strokes. The incidence of myocardial infarction and total mortality was unaffected by treatment. The results showed a much more favourable ratio of patient years of treatment to strokes prevented than, for example, the Medical Research Council Trial in younger patients: 100 patient years to prevent one stroke and 150 patient years of treatment to prevent a major or fatal stroke. This is presumably a consequence of the older age group and the higher initital blood pressure in Coope's study. See also *Atherosclerosis: Elderly and hypertension: European Working Party on Hypertension in the Elderly (EWPHE) study: Isolated systolic hypertension: Multicentre studies of clinical outcome*

Coronary arteries
The heart's blood supply is derived from the right and left coronary arteries. The right coronary artery arises from the anterior aortic sinus and passes forwards between the pulmonary trunk and the right atrium to descend in the atrio-ventricular groove, and anastomose with the left coronary artery at the posterior interventricular groove. It gives off a marginal branch and an interventricular branch. The left coronary artery arises from the left posterior aortic sinus. Passing behind and then to the left of the pulmonary trunk it reaches the atrio-ventricular groove in which it runs laterally to reach the posterior interventricular groove. Its most important branch is the anterior interventricular artery. See also *Atherosclerosis: Ischaemic heart disease: Myocardial infarction*

Coronary artery disease
This term usually refers to atherosclerosis

Coronary artery disease

affecting the coronary arteries. Coronary atherosclerosis causes angina pectoris and myocardial infarction (one of the major causes of death in the Western World). For effects of hypertension on coronary artery disease see *Ischaemic heart disease*. See also *Atherosclerosis: Myocardial infarction*

Coronary blood flow
Cardiac oxygen consumption can only be increased significantly by increasing blood flow. The latter increases when myocardial metabolism is increased. The calibre of the coronary vessels is influenced by pressure changes in the aorta, chemical factors and neural factors. See also *Coronary reflex*

Coronary reflex
'Reflex' that controls the calibre of the coronary arterioles.
Actually mediated by chemical factors and neural factors. One or more of the products of metabolism causes coronary vasodilatation. Various factors have been suggested, including oxygen lack, and increased local concentrations of carbon dioxide, hydrogen ions, potassium ions, lactic acid and others. Neural effects are mediated by the autonomic nervous system. See also *Autonomic nervous system: Coronary blood flow*

Cortex
The outer layer of an organ or other structure in the body.

Corticosteroid
Any steroid synthesized by the adrenal cortex. Divided into glucocorticoids, mineralocorticoids, and sex hormones. See also *Adrenal cortex: Glucocorticoid activity: Mineralocorticoid activity*

Corticosteroid-induced hypertension
(*also known as* Corticoid hypertension) see *Glucocorticoid-induced hypertension: Mineralocorticoid-induced hypertension*

Corticosterone
A corticosteroid which is one of the precursors of aldosterone (the immediate precursor being 18-hydroxycortico-sterone).
Corticosterone is a weak mineralo-corticoid (about 0.005 times as potent as aldosterone) and its glucocorticoid activity is about one-third that of cortisol. Corticosterone is the main corticosteroid secreted by the adrenal gland of the rat. In humans the adrenal cortex secretes about seven times as much cortisol as corticosterone. See also *Adrenal cortex: Aldosterone: Cortisol: Glucocorticoid activity: Mineralocorticoid activity*

Corticotropes
Stellate chromophobe cells of the anterior pituitary which secrete adreno-corticotrophic hormone (ACTH). Pro-opiomelanocortin is synthesized by them and then hydrolyzed to ACTH, beta-lipotrophin (β-LPH), and a small amount of beta-endorphin, all of which are secreted. See also *ACTH: Opioid peptides: Pro-opiomelanocortin*

Corticotrophin
(*also known as* Corticotropin) see *ACTH*

Corticotrophin releasing factor (CRF)
The hypothalamic peptide which stimulates release of ACTH from the anterior pituitary.
Ovine CRF has 41 amino acid residues and the human form may be similar. Intravenous ovine CRF (100 μg) causes an exaggerated response in patients with Cushing's syndrome due to pituitary hyperfunction (Cushing's disease). It may thus be helpful in diagnosis of the cause of Cushing's syndrome. See also *ACTH: Brain peptides and blood pressure control: Cushing's disease: Cushing's syndrome*

Cortisol
(*also known as* Hydrocortisone) The major glucocorticoid hormone secreted by

the human adrenal cortex. It is produced in the zona fasciculata in response to ACTH. Overproduction of cortisol leads to Cushing's syndrome. See also *ACTH: Cushing's disease: Cushing's syndrome: Glucocorticoid activity: Glucocorticoid induced hypertension*

Cortisol-binding globulin (CBG)
(*also known as* Transcortin) An alpha-globulin to which a large proportion of cortisol binds in the plasma. Cortisol binds corticosterone to a lesser degree. Bound steroid is physiologically inactive and probably functions as a circulating reservoir analogous to the situation with circulating thyroid hormones. CBG also binds to albumin to a smaller extent. CBG is synthesized in the liver and its production is increased by oestrogen. This explains why pregnant women have high total cortisol levels without features of cortisol excess. See also *Cortisol: Corticosterone*

Cortisone
A glucocorticoid secreted only in small amounts by the adrenal cortex. It is also formed in the liver as a metabolite of cortisol, which is subsequently reduced and conjugated. See also *Adrenal cortex: Cortisol: Glucocorticoid activity*

Cotransport
The movement of an ion in one direction across a membrane coupled to the movement of a different ion in the same direction. See also *Countertransport: Ion transport systems: Sodium-potassium cotransport*

Cotton-wool spots
(*also known as* Soft exudates) Small areas of infarction of retinal nerve fibres seen in severe hypertension, particularly malignant phase hypertension (Figure 42). They appear before hard exudates in the development of hypertensive retinopathy and usually disappear with control of blood pressure in 2-12 weeks. Hard

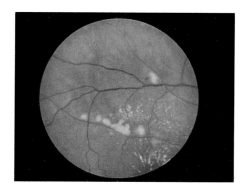

Figure 42 Cotton wool spots. In a line parallel to an attenuated vessel. A further soft exudate is seen next to the vessel nearer the top of the photograph

exudates take much longer to clear, even up to a year or more. Cotton wool spots are also found in systemic lupus erythematosus, diabetes, retinal emboli, central and branch retinal vein occlusions, and severe anaemia. See also *Hard exudates: Hypertensive retinopathy: Malignant phase hypertension*

Countertransport
The movement of an ion in one direction across a membrane coupled to the movement of a different ion in the opposite direction. See also *Cotransport: Ion transport systems: Sodium-hydrogen ion countertransport: Sodium-lithium countertransport*

Creatinine
An end-product of creatine metabolism. Its endogenous production correlates with muscle mass, and tends to be constant for a given individual. Plasma or serum concentration gives an estimate of glomerular filtration but creatinine clearance is more accurate if complete urine collections are achieved. Measurements of serum creatine concentrations are useful for serial monitoring of renal function. See also *Creatinine clearance*

Creatinine clearance

Measurement which approximates to glomerular filtration rate (GFR).
The ideal substance for the estimation of GFR would be freely filtered at the glomerulus, and not secreted, reabsorbed, catabolized, or synthesized. Creatinine is freely filtered, but is also secreted by the proximal tubule. Creatinine clearance, therefore, usually overestimates GFR. Colorimetric measurements of plasma creatinine tend to overestimate the concentration due to the presence of noncreatinine chromogens and this may counterbalance the effect of renal secretion. In moderate renal failure creatinine secretion may rise until GFR falls below 10 ml / min so that creatinine clearance further overestimates GFR. In advanced renal failure, creatinine clearance approximately equals GFR.
Creatinine clearance = UV/ P where
U = urinary creatinine concentration,
V = urinary production rate in ml / min and
P = plasma creatinine concentration.

Table 13 Major clinical features of Cushing's syndrome

Obesity, usually in a truncal distribution (Figure 43a) often with a moon face (Figure 43b), buffalo hump and protuberant abdomen

Purple abdominal striae (see Figure 43a) and purpura (42%)

Hypertension (75%)

Oedema (20%)

Hirsutism (30%)

Muscle weakness and atrophy (36%) usually affecting the proximal limb muscles (Fig.43c)

Psychiatric disturbance with psychosis (6%)

Irregular menstruation, particularly oligomenorrhoea (72%)

Osteoporosis (58%) with back pain

Impaired glucose tolerance (94%)

Growth retardation in children

Strictly speaking, this should be corrected to average body surface area (1.73 m^2).
See also *Body surface area nomogram: Chronic renal failure: Glomerular filtration rate: Inulin clearance*

CRF
Corticotrophin releasing factor

Cushing's disease
(Harvey Williams Cushing, U.S. neurosurgeon, 1869-1939)
Cushing's syndrome due to hypothalamic-pituitary dysfunction. Accounts for 70% of cases of the syndrome when it is not iatrogenic. Excess production of ACTH causes bilateral adrenal cortical hyperplasia. Most cases are associated with pituitary adenomas which secrete

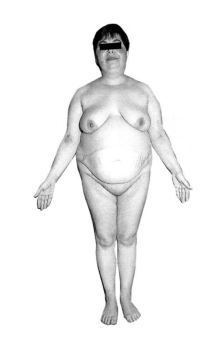

Figure 43(a) Cushing's syndrome. Due to hypothalamic-pituitary dysfunction (Cushing's disease). Note the truncal obesity and abdominal striae

excessive ACTH. This oversecretion probably results from abnormal stimulation by corticotrophin releasing factor. Evidence for a hypothalamic origin for hypersecretion of pituitary ACTH includes the following:

ACTH release in the disease is not autonomous; it can be inhibited by sufficient glucocorticoid. ACTH secretion can also be affected by various agents, for example, bromocriptine, acting upon central nervous system neurotransmission;

These patients often have other evidence of hypothalamic dysfunction;

Some patients have persistent Cushing's syndrome after successful removal of a pituitary adenoma.

For clinical features, diagnosis and treatment see Cushing's syndrome and Tables 13 and 15. See also *ACTH: Adrenal hyperplasia: Bromocriptine: Corticotrophin releasing factor: Hyperplasia: Hypothalamus: Pituitary gland*

Cushing's law
Increase of intracranial pressure causes increase of systemic arterial blood pressure to a point slightly above the pressure exerted on the medulla. See also *Cushing's reflex*

Cushing's reflex
When intracranial pressure is increased the blood supply to the vasomotor centre is impaired and local hypoxia and hypercapnia increase its discharge. This

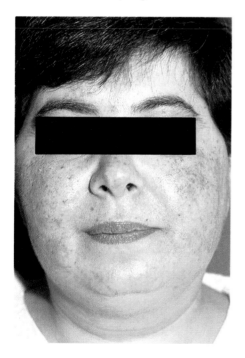

Figure 43(b) Moon face in Cushing's disease

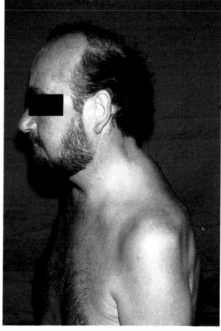

Figure 43(c) Muscle wasting in Cushing's syndrome due to ectopic ACTH secretion

Cushing's reflex

causes increased arterial blood pressure which tends to restore the blood flow to the medulla. The rise in blood pressure is accompanied by a baroreceptor-mediated reflex bradycardia. See also *Baroreceptors: Cardioinhibitory centre: Intracranial hypertension: Vasomotor centre*

Cushing's syndrome

The syndrome caused by excessive glucocorticoid in the form of cortisol or therapeutically administered steroids. Apart from iatrogenic disease, hypo-thalamic-pituitary dysfunction is the most common cause. Ectopic ACTH production by various tumours and cortisol production by adrenal neoplasms each make up 15% of the non-iatrogenic cases. The most common source of ectopic ACTH production is small cell (oat cell) carcinoma of the bronchus. Other tumours include carcinoids, medullary thyroid carcinoma, pancreatic islet cell tumours, phaeochromocytomas, ganglioneuromas, malignant melanomas and carcinoma of the prostate.

Adrenal cortical tumours causing Cushing's syndrome are usually single and may be benign (adenomas) or malignant (carcinomas). There may be associated virilization. The main feature distinguishing these cases from those due to hypothalamic-pituitary dysfunction and ectopic ACTH production is suppression of pituitary ACTH production with often undetectable plasma concentrations.

Hypertension

Hypertension in Cushing's syndrome may be severe and cause increasing morbidity if left untreated. It may persist despite removal of the cause. Table 14 compares the clinical and laboratory features of Cushing's disease and ectopic ACTH

Table 14 Ectopic ACTH secretion compared with Cushing's disease

		Ectopic ACTH syndrome	
	Cushing's Disease	Oat cell carcinoma	Carcinoid tumours
Sex	Mostly female	Mostly male	Equal
Pigmentation	Uncommon	Common	Sometimes
Speed of onset	Slow	Rapid	Slow
Oedema	Rare	Common	Rare
Weight loss	Rare	Common	Rare
Clinical course	Years	Days to weeks	Years
Cause of death	Hypertension, infection	Carcinoma	Carcinoma or cardiovascular
K <3.3 mmol/ litre	Unusual	Usual	Usual
HCO_3<30 mmol/ litre	Unusual	Usual	Usual
Diabetic glucose tolerance test	Sometimes	Usual	Usual
Plasma ACTH over 200 pg/ ml	Very unusual	Usual	Common
Plasma cortisol over 1000 nmol/ litre (36µg/ 100ml)	Very unusual	Usual	Sometimes but often < 800 nmol/ litre (30 µg/100ml)
Response to dexamethasone 8 mg/ day	Usual	Very rare	Rare
Response to metyrapone	Marked	Very rare	Sometimes

production. Diagnosis of the cause of Cushing's syndrome is summarized by Table 15.

Treatment

Treatment of Cushing's disease is often by hypophysectomy especially trans-sphenoidal, by an experienced surgeon. Pituitary irradiation has been used for many years using various techniques. Metyrapone can also be used to lower plasma cortisol levels. Ectopic ACTH production is treated by resection of the responsible lesion where possible or treatment with metyrapone. Adrenocortical adenomas or carcinomas are resected as fully as possible. See also *Cushing's disease: Glucocorticoid-induced hypertension :* and *table 13*

Cyclic adenosine $3',5'$-monophosphate (cAMP)

see *Adenosine $3',5'$-cyclic phosphate*

Table 15 Cushing's syndrome: Diagnostic tests

(a) Screening tests
(1) Overnight dexamethasone suppression test (see Dexamethasone suppression tests)
(2) Urinary free cortisol: expressed either as µg/day or as a urinary cortisol/creatinine ratio. Normal values depend on method used to measure the urinary cortisol

(b) Definitive tests
Confirming hypersecretion of cortisol
(1) Plasma cortisol diurnal rhythm: plasma concentrations measured at 09.00h and 24.00h may show loss of the normal diurnal rhythm, and the values should be high compared to the respective reference ranges. However, increased midnight cortisol concentration can be due to stress or depression.
(2) Urinary free cortisol: repeated measurements may be needed especially if hypersecretion of cortisol is intermittent.
(3) Plasma cortisol response to hypoglycaemia: may be useful in distinguishing Cushing's syndrome from hypercortisolaemia due to depression. Only in the former case will the cortisol response to adequate hypoglycaemia (<2.2 mmol/1) be reduced.

Indicating cause of hypersecretion of cortisol
(1) Plasma ACTH diurnal rhythm: undetectable ACTH suggests a primary adrenal lesion (see text) provided the value is not falsely low because of careless processing of plasma. Very high values suggest ectopic ACTH production (see Table 14). In Cushing's disease the 09.00h value may be normal, but the midnight value is usually high.
(2) Prolonged dexamethasone suppression test (see Dexamethasone suppression tests)
(3) Metyrapone test (see Metyrapone test): Found useful by some in differentiating between Cushing's disease and ectopic ACTH production.
(4) Radiological investigation:
(a) Lateral skull x-ray may show enlargement of the pituitary fossa in Cushing's disease.
(b) Chest radiograph may demonstrate bronchogenic carcinoma or more rarely a bronchial carcinoid.
(c) Computed tomographic scanning may show a unilateral adrenocortical neoplasm or bilateral adrenal hyperplasia in Cushing's disease.
(d) Adrenal scintigraphy may also be useful.
(e) Adrenal venography and adrenal venous sampling are reserved for difficult cases.

Cyclic guanosine 3′, 5′-monophosphate

Cyclic guanosine 3′,5′-monophosphate
see *Guanosine 3′,5′-cyclic phosphate*

Cyclohexanehexol
see *Inositol*

Cyclo-oxygenase
An enzyme involved in the synthesis of
prostaglandins. See also *Prostaglandins*

Cyclopenthiazide
A thiazide diuretic used in the treatment of
hypertension. See also *Thiazide diuretics*

Cyclothiazide
A thiazide diuretic used in the treatment of
hypertension. See also *Thiazide diuretics*

D

Dahl rats
(Lewis K Dahl, U.S. physician, 1914–1975)
Two strains of rat developed by selective
inbreeding of Sprague-Dawley rats. Dahl
salt-sensitive (DS) rats are susceptible to
development of hypertension on a high salt
diet, while in the salt-resistant (DR) strain,
blood pressure is insensitive to salt.
Later observations by Dahl suggested
increased pressor responsiveness to a
wide range of noxious stimuli in the
'sensitive strain' and the specificity of 'salt
sensitivity' is doubtful. Cross-circulation
studies suggest that a circulating factor
is responsible for hypertension in the
DS strain (Figure 44). Salt-sensitivity can
be produced in a DR rat by linking its
circulation with that of a DS rat. Hypertension can also be conferred on a DR rat
by transplanting into it a kidney from a
DS rat (Figure 44). There are similarities
between DS rats and Milan hypertensive
rats, but pressor sensitivity to salt is much
greater in the DS strain. See also *Bianchi-
Milan spontaneously hypertensive rats:
Rat strains in hypertension research*

Debrisoquine
An adrenergic neurone blocker with
haemodynamic effects similar to
guanethidine and bretylium, but having
shorter duration of action. Little used in
modern practice.

Dehydroepiandrosterone (DHEA)
A weakly androgenic steroid hormone
secreted by the adrenal cortex in response
to ACTH which is of little importance
except when secreted in grossly excessive
amounts, in, for example, virilizing
congenital adrenal hyperplasia. DHEA is
the major precursor of the urinary 17-
ketosteroids.

11-Deoxycorticosterone (DOC)
An adrenocortical steroid with significant
mineralocorticoid activity (however, only
about 3% of the activity of aldosterone).
It is normally secreted in similar
amounts to aldosterone, and may cause
hypertension if secreted in greatly
increased amounts as in some forms of
congenital adrenal hyperplasia (see 11 β-
hydroxylase deficiency, 17 α-hydroxylase
deficiency). See also *Congenital adrenal
hyperplasia*

Deoxycorticosterone acetate (DOCA)
An acetate of deoxycorticosterone (see
above) which is used with sodium chloride
to induce hypertension in the rat (DOCA-
salt hypertension). Usually unilateral
nephrectomy is also carried out. This is
used as an experimental model of
mineralocorticoid hypertension. See also
Mineralocorticoid-induced hypertension

11-Deoxycortisol
The immediate precursor of cortisol in
adrenal steroid synthesis (see Figure 5).
Plasma levels may increase with ineffi-
ciency of the enzyme 11 β-hydroxylase, for
example, in a form of congenital adrenal
hyperplasia, in carcinomatous adrenals,
and with metyrapone treatment. Normally,
it has little biological activity.

Depolarization
The cells of excitable tissues (nerve and
muscle) have an electrical potential
difference across their cell membranes
(resting membrane potential is approximately -70 to -90 mV). Electrical
impulses can be transmitted along these
cell membranes by propagation of a region
of depolarization where the membrane
potential 'changes sign' and becomes
positive. This change results from
alterations in ion fluxes across the plasma
membrane. The term 'action potential'
includes the whole sequence from the
resting state through depolarization and
back to the resting state again. In smooth
muscle the membrane potential has no

Depolarization

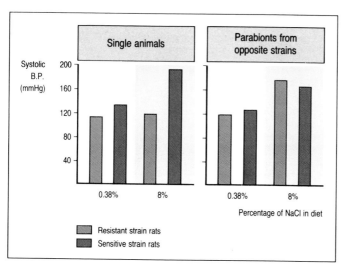

Figure 44a Dahl rats
When the circulation of a Dahl salt-sensitive rat is connected to that of a salt-resistant rat, or vice versa, the blood pressure differences between the two strains disappear.

true resting value, being relatively low when the muscle is very active and higher when it is relatively inactive. See also *Tone: Vascular smooth muscle*

Depression
Mood characterized by dejection and pessimism. Hypertension and mental depression may be linked in at least three ways: certain antihypertensive drugs may cause depression, some antidepressant drugs may interact with certain antihypertensive drugs, and reactive depression and anxiety may be caused by frequent attendance at hypertension clinics. Of the older antihypertensive agents reserpine is the drug classically associated with depression. This was thought to have caused suicide in some cases, but with currently used lower doses the association is less clear. Alpha-methyldopa may also cause depression, as may administration of clonidine or even beta-adrenergic receptor blocking drugs, although the association with the latter group of drugs is very uncommon. The therapeutic effect of guanethidine, alpha-methyldopa and possibly clonidine is antagonized by tricyclic antidepressant

drugs. However, these three anti-hypertensive drugs are less frequently used now and this interaction should not be a great problem. Depression can cause increased plasma concentrations of cortisol requiring differentiation from Cushing's syndrome. See also *Alpha-methyldopa: Beta-adrenergic receptor blocking drugs: Clonidine: Guanethidine: Reserpine*

Des-angiotensin I renin substrate
The protein remaining after the removal of the angiotensin I sequence from the N-terminal portion of angiotensinogen (renin substrate). (See Figure 13)

Des-aspartyl angiotensin
Des-aspartyl angiotensin I is a minor intermediate in the pathway from angiotensin I to angiotensin III (see Figure 13). It has little biological activity. Des-aspartyl angiotensin II is another name for angiotensin III.

Desmopressin
(*also known as* 1-(3-Mercaptopropionic acid)-8-D-arginine vasopressin)
A synthetic analogue of arginine

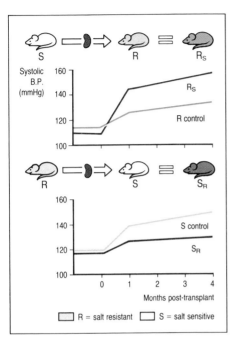

Figure 44b Dahl rats. Renal cross-transplantation in Dahl rats: grafting of a kidney from a salt-sensitive (DS) rat into a nephrectomized salt-resistant rat produces hypertension whereas transplantation of a kidney from a D R rat into a nephrectomized DS rat has the opposite effect.

vasopressin used in the treatment of diabetes insipidus. See also *Antidiuretic hormone: Diabetes insipidus*

Dexamethasone
A synthetic glucocorticoid analogue which is 25 times more potent than cortisol in terms of anti-inflammatory effect.

Dexamethasone-suppressible aldosteronism
(*also known as* Glucocorticoid-remediable aldosteronism) A rare form of primary aldosteronism.
Patients usually present with hypertension, hypokalaemia, raised plasma

aldosterone concentration, and low plasma renin activity, but usually administration of glucocorticoids reverses the abnormalities within two weeks (Figure 45). There appears to be a major influence of ACTH on aldosterone secretion in this group of patients. Surgical exploration reveals zona glomerulosa hyperplasia. The disease may be familial, apparently with autosomal dominant transmission. The pathogenesis of the condition remains unclear. See also *Aldosteronism: Conn's syndrome: Hypokalaemia: Idiopathic aldosteronism: Mineralocorticoid-induced hypertension*

Dexamethasone suppression tests
The overnight dexamethasone suppression test is used to diagnose Cushing's syndrome. A single 2 mg dose is given orally at 23.00 hours. If plasma cortisol concentration at 08.00 hours next morning is greater than 200 nmol / l this suggests the presence of Cushing's syndrome. The prolonged dexamethasone suppression test is used to determine the cause of Cushing's syndrome. Plasma cortisol (at 08.00–09.00 h) and urinary metabolites are measured before and during the first two days' treatment with dexamethasone 0.5 mg qds. This will suppress cortisol in normal subjects and some patients with Cushing's disease. In response to a further two days of dexamethasone 2 mg qds, suppression is seen in most other patients with Cushing's disease. No suppression is seen with ectopic ACTH production and with primary adrenal lesions. See also *Dexamethasone-suppressible aldosteronism*

Diabetes insipidus (DI)
A rare metabolic disorder in which polyuria results from either deficiency of antidiuretic hormone (cranial DI) or renal resistance to the action of antidiuretic hormone (nephrogenic DI).
In cranial DI, urine output ranges from 2–15 litres per day. Plasma antidiuretic hormone concentration is low and

Diabetes insipidus

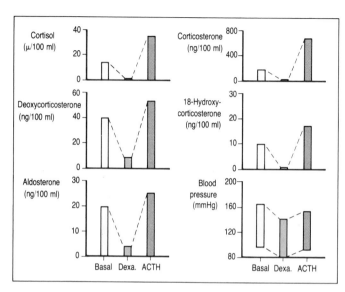

Figure 45 Dexamethasone-suppressible aldosteronism. Plasma corticosteroid concentrations and blood pressure in a patient with dexamethasone-suppressible aldosteronism untreated (Basal); after four days of oral dexamethasone 2 mg daily (Dexa); and after seven days of ACTH 2 mg/day intramuscularly (ACTH).

patients rely on thirst to maintain normal plasma osmolality. Most cases fall into the idiopathic category. Diagnosis can be made by measuring plasma and urine osmolality in a water deprivation test (urine osmolality fails to increase with that of plasma, and this can be corrected with exogenous antidiuretic hormone). Treatment is by means of intranasal desmopressin. In nephrogenic DI, hypotonic urine during a water deprivation test fails to respond to exogenous antidiuretic hormone. Treatment is unsatisfactory, though thiazide diuretics may be helpful. See also *Antidiuretic hormone: Desmopressin: Water deprivation test*

Diabetes mellitus (DM)
A syndrome characterized by diminished glucose tolerance due to deficiency or diminished effectiveness of insulin, which may be divided into primary diabetes and secondary diabetes.
Classification In the latter case the diabetes is secondary to another disease process. Primary diabetes can be

subdivided into Type I (insulin-dependent) and Type II (non-insulin dependent). In the vast majority of patients with both hypertension and diabetes mellitus, the latter is of the primary type. There are, in fact, interesting parallels between essential hypertension, Type II diabetes mellitus and obesity. These conditions are also associated with increased levels of vascular growth factors (including either insulin or insulin-like growth factor I) and an increased risk of atherosclerotic diseases such as ischaemic heart disease. In view of this increased risk, control of blood pressure is particularly important in hypertensive diabetics. Secondary diabetes or impaired glucose tolerance may be produced by some causes of secondary hypertension, particularly Cushing's syndrome and phaeo-chromocytoma, and sometimes Conn's syndrome.
Antihypertensive drugs and diabetes
Diuretic drugs, particularly thiazides, may induce mild glucose intolerance. This can be overcome in Type I diabetics by increasing their insulin dosage, but

thiazides are not recommended for Type II diabetics, being treated with diet or oral hypoglycaemic drugs. Beta-adrenergic receptor blocking drugs inhibit the normal metabolic response to, and may mask the symptoms of hypoglycaemia. They should be avoided if possible in Type I diabetics, especially if diabetic control is variable. Vasodilators and alpha-methyldopa may be used safely in diabetics as may calcium antagonists and angiotensin I converting enzyme inhibitors. See also *Growth factors: Insulin and insulin-like growth factors: Obesity and hypertension*

Diabetic nephropathy
Term used to denote renal disease caused by diabetes mellitus. It is associated with diabetic microangiopathy (small blood vessel disease), and retinopathy occurs in nearly all patients with diabetic nephropathy.
Pathological and clinical features The disease is characterized by glomerulosclerosis, in which there is thickening of the basement membrane and enlargement of the mesangium. Early diabetic nephropathy is indicated by mild proteinuria. Later heavier proteinuria may be found and nephrotic syndrome and renal failure may develop. Functionally, renal failure is preceded by glomerular

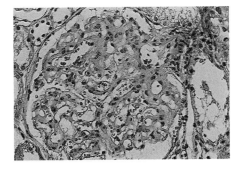

Figure 46 Diabetic nephropathy. The kidney in human diabetes: diffuse glomerulo-sclerosis showing diffuse, uneven thickening of the capillary wall.

hyperfiltration, which is believed to be an important factor in subsequent nephron loss. Hypertension may not develop until a late stage.
Treatment Diabetic nephropathy may be prevented or its progression slowed by meticulous diabetic control, careful control of coexistent hypertension, and stopping cigarette smoking. End-stage renal failure may result from diabetic nephropathy, and continuous ambulatory peritoneal dialysis is often used in these patients. Insulin may be administered via the dialysis fluid. (Figure 46) See also *Chronic renal failure: Renal disease causing hypertension*

Diacylglycerol (DG)
see *Inositol lipid metabolism*

Dialysis
The technique used in the management of end-stage renal failure in which the solute content of the blood is altered by allowing blood to exchange solute with fluid on the other side of a dialysis membrane, either synthetic, as in haemodialysis, or biological (the peritoneal membrane in peritoneal dialysis).
Renal dialysis is usually started for chronic renal failure when serum creatinine concentration is 1000-1200 μmol / l, but it is sometimes indicated earlier on symptomatic grounds. Hypertension in most patients with end-stage renal failure can be controlled by salt and water depletion (by dialysis), but about 10% will need continued antihypertensive medication. Bilateral nephrectomy is seldom, if ever, necessary since the advent of angiotensin I converting enzyme inhibitors. See also *Bilateral nephrectomy: Chronic renal failure*

Diapamide
A diuretic with antihypertensive properties. See also *Diuretics*

Diastole
The period in the cardiac contraction cycle

97

Diastole

when all four chambers of the heart are relaxed. See also *Systole*

Diastolic blood pressure

Pressure exerted by blood in the arterial tree during diastole. See also *Arterial blood pressure*

Diazoxide

A powerful vasodilator drug used primarily for hypertensive emergencies (for example, hypertensive encephalopathy or dissecting aortic aneurysm). Unlike nitroprusside, it does not have much effect on venous capacitance, and can cause marked sodium and water retention, requiring the use of potent diuretics. Given intravenously by infusion it is less likely to cause severe hypotension than if it is given as a bolus. Side-effects include hyperglycaemia, renal impairment, hirsutism, and hypersensitivity reactions. See also *Dissecting aortic aneurysm: Hypertensive encephalopathy: Vasodilators*

Dichloroisoprenaline

(*also known as* DCI: Dichloroisoproterenol) The first drug to produce selective beta-adrenergic antagonism. It is not used clinically in man because of its prominent β-adrenergic (partial agonist) stimulant action. See also *Agonist: Antagonist*

Dichloroisoproterenol

Synonym for dichloroisoprenaline.

Diet and hypertension

Numerous dietary types or dietary components have been implicated in the aetiology of essential hypertension (Table 16). It has been suggested that modification of various aspects of the diet may have a role in non-drug treatment of hypertension. Much of the information implying associations between dietary components and hypertension comes from epidemiological surveys in which dietary habits are compared in populations with different blood pressure levels (see for example *High sodium, high blood pressure populations: Low sodium, low blood pressure populations*). However, the populations compared often differ in respects other than diet and this makes the analysis of the situation difficult. Another experimental approach which has been used in the study of the relationship between diet and hypertension is assessment of the antihypertensive effect of altering dietary composition, for example, lowering sodium intake or increasing potassium intake. See also *Alcohol: Cadmium: Calcium: Lead: Magnesium: Obesity and hypertension: Vegetarian diet*

Dietary sodium and potassium in hypertension

(special contribution from Dr Graham Watt, Greater Glasgow Health Board Glasgow, Scotland) In clinical practice, the main interest in studying the effect of altering intakes of dietary sodium and potassium has been related to the possibility of managing hypertensive patients without drugs. Since initial blood pressure levels are known to fall with repeated measurement, it should be recognized that uncontrolled observations of the effect of dietary measures in individual patients provide a very unreliable guide to the efficacy of these measures. Since alterations in diet may have social and cost implications for patients, it behoves clinicians to base their advice on double-blind, randomized controlled clinical trials, whenever possible.

Dietary sodium
None of the studies of reducing sodium intake in hypertensive patients which have met the criteria above have described the initial blood pressures of the patients in a way which permits ready extrapolation to clinical practice. However, it is generally agreed that

sodium restriction does lower blood pressure by about 6 / 4 mmHg in patients with blood pressures which are high enough to warrant drug treatment - say, over 100 mmHg diastolic phase 5. In the range 90-99 mmHg, reducing sodium intake appears to have little or no effect on blood pressure. Older patients may be more susceptible to reductions in sodium intake. Sodium restriction therefore seems to be of limited use in those who are most eligible for non-pharmacological treatment - namely, young patients with mild hypertension. The contribution of a reduction in sodium intake may therefore be to reduce the requirement for drugs, rather than to avoid the need for drug treatment. By virtue of their method of action, some drugs (for example, angiotensin I converting enzyme inhibitors) may exhibit a synergistic effect in association with reducing sodium intake.

Advice to reduce sodium intake should not take precedence over other measures which are known to reduce blood pressure such as maintenance of ideal body weight and moderation of alcohol intake, nor advice directed towards the prevention of coronary artery disease such as stopping smoking and reducing the intake of saturated fat.

The only reliable method of measuring sodium intake, or changes in sodium intake during sodium restriction is to measure serial 24-hour urinary excretion. Mean sodium intakes in western populations range from about 120 mmol to about 300 mmol per day. Within each population however there is also a very wide range of intakes. Individuals also vary widely in their intake from day to day. The levels achieved by patients in clinical trials are in the range 80-100 mmol per day.

Upwards of 70% of dietary intake comes from sodium which is added to food by manufacturers. Major changes in intake therefore require a reduction in high sodium foodstuffs. The nutritional

Table 16 Diet and hypertension

Dietary component	Direction of association
Sodium	Direct
Potassium	Inverse
Calcium	Inverse
Magnesium	Inverse
Protein	Direct
Saturated fat	Direct
Unsaturated fat	Inverse
Dietary fibre	Inverse
Pantothenic acid	Inverse
Tyrosine	Inverse
Selenium	Inverse
Cadmium	Direct
Lead	Direct
Copper	Direct
Zinc	Direct

Other dietary factors

Coffee	Equivocal
Alcohol	Direct
High calorie intake	Direct
Vegetarian diet	Inverse

consequences of such changes are largely unstudied. Concerted action to reduce the sodium content of processed foods would increase the feasibility of sodium restriction, and avoid other nutritional consequences.

Dietary potassium
Potassium intakes in western countries range from about 40 to 80 mmol per day. Some, but not all, double-blind, randomized controlled trials of the effect

of increasing potassium intake by 60-100 mmol per day show a small hypotensive effect of 3-4 mmHg. Potassium supplements are unpalatable, and it is difficult to achieve this degree of potassium loading by purely dietary means. For this reason, and also because of the possibility of harming patients with unsuspected renal disease, there has been less enthusiasm for altering the potassium intakes of hypertensive patients. See also *Diet and hypertension: High sodium, high blood pressure populations: Low sodium, low blood pressure populations*

Digital subtraction angiography
(*also know as* Digital vascular imaging) Using computer processing to improve resolution, this radiological technique allows images to be obtained of arteries, for example, renal arteries, following injection of contrast medium into a vein, usually the superior vena cava (via a central venous pressure line). For examples of digital subtraction angiograms see Figures 12 and 28

Digitalis
Term applied to the group of drugs known also as the cardiac glycosides.
Each glycoside consists of a part called the aglycone and from one to four molecules of sugar. Members of the group include digoxin and ouabain. The cardiac glycosides have a positive inotropic effect which results from inhibition by the drug of the sodium-potassium adenosine triphosphatase in cardiac muscle cells. This inhibition causes increased intracellular calcium concentration which is responsible for the effect on muscle contraction.
The positive inotropic effect of digoxin is the reason for its use in the treatment of cardiac failure, although there is debate as to whether this beneficial action is maintained in the long term. The cardiac glycosides also have effects on the conducting system of the heart, and digoxin is widely used to reduce the ventricular rate in patients with atrial fibrillation.
Digoxin-like drugs may also exhibit a mild diuretic action which is not likely to be observed in the presence of other more powerful diuretic agents. Overdosage of digoxin produces numerous, often serious, adverse effects and careful choice of dose is important, particularly if renal function is impaired.

Digitalis-like natriuretic factor
Administration of digitalis leads to inhibition of the sodium-potassium adenosine triphosphatase. In vascular smooth muscle this enhances depolarization and vasoconstriction, while in the renal tubules there is natriuresis caused by reduced tubular sodium reabsorption. Evidence has been found of an endogenous digitalis-like substance or substances in humans given a saline infusion, in patients with essential hypertension, and in normotensive subjects with a family history of hypertension.
The natriuretic factor (or hormone) inhibits the sodium-potassium adenosine triphosphatase and also antagonizes binding of ouabain to the digitalis binding site on the red blood cells. The factor that appears after acute volume expansion appears to be a heat-stable molecule bound to a protein. Its origin is unclear. Evidence suggests the presence of digitalis-like natriuretic factor in patients with acromegaly, in whom plasma volume is expanded. The activity of the factor in plasma correlates inversely with plasma renin activity and directly with plasma volume and arterial pressure.
Some investigators consider that the natriuretic factor may be responsible for raised blood pressure in low renin hypertension. They postulate that impaired renal sodium excretion causes increased intravascular volume which triggers release of the natriuretic substance. The latter would then cause natriuresis, tending to restore intravascular volume

to normal, but would also cause hypertension due to vasoconstriction. Despite many years of investigation the natriuretic substance remains a subject of controversy and its precise nature is unknown. See also *Blaustein hypothesis: Cell sodium hypothesis: Ion transport systems*

Digoxin
see *Digitalis: Digitalis-like natriuretic factor*

Dihydralazine (dihydrallazine)
A vasodilator antihypertensive drug related to hydralazine.

Dihydroergotamine
Drug related to ergotamine used in the treatment of orthostatic hypotension because of its powerful and relatively selective vasoconstrictor effect on the capacitance vessels (the venous side of the circulation). This probably results from stimulation of alpha-adrenergic receptors. It has been shown to be effective, at least in the short term, when given parenterally for postural hypotension, but has potentially serious side-effects and is poorly absorbed when taken orally. See also *Orthostatic hypotension*

Dihydropyridines
One of the main groups of calcium antagonists. It includes drugs such as nifedipine, nitrendipine, nicardipine, nimodipine and felodipine (see individual entries).

3,4-Dihydroxymandelic acid (DOMA)
A metabolite of adrenaline and noradrenaline formed from 3,4-dihydroxyphenylglycolaldehyde (DOPGAL) in a reaction catalyzed by aldehyde dehydrogenase (aldehyde oxidase). See also *Catecholamine metabolites*

3,4-Dihydroxymandelic aldehyde
Synonym for 3,4-dihydroxyphenylglycolaldehyde.

3,4-Dihydroxyphenylacetic acid (DOPAC)
A metabolite of dopamine formed in a reaction catalyzed by monoamine oxidase.

Dihydroxyphenylalanine (DOPA)
An intermediate in the synthesis of dopamine, noradrenaline and adrenaline from tyrosine.

Dihydroxyphenylalanine decarboxylase
(*also known as* DOPA decarboxylase)
Enzyme which catalyzes the conversion of dihydroxyphenylalanine (DOPA) to dopamine. DOPA decarboxylase seems to be identical to the enzyme which catalyzes formation of 5-hydroxytryptamine (serotonin) from 5-hydroxytryptophan. The term L-aromatic amino acid decarboxylase may be preferable.

Dihydroxyphenylethylamine
Synonym (little used) for dopamine.

3,4-Dihydroxyphenylethylene glycol (DOPEG)
A metabolite of noradrenaline and adrenaline formed from 3,4-dihydroxyphenylglycolaldehyde (DOPGAL) in a reaction catalyzed by alcohol dehydrogenase (aldehyde reductase). See also *Catecholamine metabolites*

3,4-Dihydroxyphenylglycolaldehyde
(*also known as* DOPGAL: 3,4-Dihydroxymandelic aldehyde) A metabolite of noradrenaline and adrenaline formed in a reaction catalyzed by monoamine oxidase. See also *Catecholamine metabolites*

5,6-Dihydroxytryptamine (5,6-DHT)
An analogue of 5-hydroxytryptamine (serotonin). It is neurotoxic and preferentially destroys 5-hydroxytryptamine-containing neurones. It has been used to study the possible role of central 5-hydroxytryptamine in causing

5,6-Dihydroxytryptamine

hypertension in various experimental models: for example, centrally administered 5,6-DHT reduces sinoaortic baroreceptor denervation hypertension. See also *5-Hydroxytryptamine: Sinoaortic baroreceptor denervation*

Diltiazem

A calcium antagonist of the benzothiazepine class which has been shown to lower blood pressure in rats and humans, but to date has been less used for hypertension than nifedipine or verapamil. Currently used more for the prophylaxis and treatment of angina pectoris. Pharmacological properties *in vivo* are summarized in Table 9. Diltiazem slows atrioventricular conduction, but to a lesser extent than verapamil. Significant negative inotropic effect is rare, but because of the risk of bradycardia, diltiazem should be used with caution in conjunction with beta-adrenergic receptor blocking drugs. Most studies show a low frequency of side-effects, but these have included headaches, oedema and rashes.

Dipeptidyl carboxypeptidase

see *Angiotensin I converting enzyme*

Dipyridamole

Used in combination with aspirin this antiplatelet drug prolongs the survival of platelets in patients with thrombotic diseases. It appears to inhibit cyclic nucleotide phosphodiesterase activity in the platelet and potentiates the effect of prostacyclin. When combined with aspirin it has been recommended for the prevention of thrombosis or embolism in patients with previous myocardial infarction, in patients who have had balloon angioplasty of a stenosed artery, and in patients with prosthetic heart valves. Efficacy is doubtful. See also *Aspirin*

Direct Coomb's test

(RRA Coombs, English physician and immunologist, born 1921) This is an immunological test for autoimmune haemolysis, for example, that induced by alpha-methyldopa. After two to three months on this drug 5–10% of patients will have a positive test caused by the presence of immunoglobulin G directed against components of the Rh complex locus. Complement is almost never fixed. In most patients little if any haemolysis occurs but there is a significant amount in a minority associated with spherocytosis and splenomegaly. Antibody usually disappears within two to three months of stopping the drug. See also *Alpha-methyldopa*

Direct vasodilators

see *Vasodilators*

Dissecting aortic aneurysm

An aneurysm resulting from an intimal tear, or an intramural haemorrhage which ruptures into the aortic lumen. It is usually associated with cystic medial necrosis, for example, in Marfan's and Ehlers-Danlos syndromes. The tear occurs either in the ascending aorta or at the junction of the arch and the descending aorta, and may cause aortic regurgitation, myocardial ischaemia, cardiac tamponade, left haemothorax or compromise any of the aortic branches. It usually presents with very severe interscapular pain. The major part of medical treatment is aimed at lowering the blood pressure, if raised, for example, using intravenous nitroprusside. Definitive treatment is surgical. See also *Nitroprusside*

Diuretics

Drugs which increase the volume of urine. The main diuretics used in the treatment of hypertension can be divided into thiazides, loop diuretics, and potassium-sparing diuretics. Thiazides are common first line drugs for mild hypertension although concern has been voiced about potentially adverse effects on serum lipid, glucose, potassium and uric acid concentrations.

The mechanism of action in lowering blood pressure is not clear, but appears to depend on producing a negative sodium balance. The long-term effect is reduction of peripheral resistance. Most thiazides become ineffective with significantly impaired renal function and in this situation a switch to a loop diuretic would be advisable. Potassium-sparing diuretics may be used to correct hypokalaemia caused by other diuretics or may be used in the medical treatment of Conn's syndrome and idiopathic aldosteronism. See also *Loop diuretics: Potassium-sparing diuretics: Thiazide diuretics*

Diurnal variation in blood pressure
It is well-established that blood pressure tends to rise from early morning to a maximum between 17.00 and 19.00 h. During sleep, blood pressure readings made by indirect methods tend to fall. This is confirmed by measurements made directly using intra-arterial cannulae which show a fall in systolic, diastolic and mean arterial pressure during sleep, and cardiac rate also falls. Although this applies in hypertensive as well as normotensive subjects, it has been found by some researchers that patients with malignant phase hypertension have little fall in blood pressure during sleep. In both normotensive and hypertensive subjects the rise in blood pressure during the day seems to be gradual, but blood pressure falls rapidly during the first few hours of sleep. See also *Ambulatory blood pressure monitoring: Measurement of blood pressure: Seasonal variation in blood pressure*

Dobutamine
A drug, related to dopamine, which acts as a beta$_1$-adrenergic agonist. By this means it produces a positive inotropic effect on the heart, but it has little positive chronotropic effect at normal doses. Dobutamine does not act on dopaminergic receptors but infusion causes increased cardiac output with little effect on heart rate or peri-

pheral resistance. The drug is used in the treatment of cardiogenic and septic shock.

DOCA-salt hypertensive rats
see *Deoxycorticosterone acetate*

DOPA
see *Dihydroxyphenylalanine*

DOPA decarboxylase
see *Dihydroxyphenylalanine decarboxylase*

DOPAC
see *3,4-Dihydroxyphenylacetic acid*

Dopamine
A catecholamine which is a precursor of both adrenaline and noradrenaline. It is secreted in small amounts by the human adrenal medulla and acts as an important neurotransmitter in the central nervous system. The physiological function of circulating dopamine is unknown. The cardiovascular effects of intravenous infusion are complex. Stimulation of peripheral dopamine 1 receptors causes vasodilatation especially in the renal, coronary, mesenteric and cerebral vascular beds. Stimulation of peripheral dopamine 2 receptors on the nerve endings of post-ganglionic sympathetic neurones inhibits the release of noradrenaline. Dopamine can also act as an agonist at beta$_1$-receptors, stimulating the heart and alpha-receptors, causing vasoconstriction. The net effects of intravenous infusion at low or intermediate doses are usually increased systolic and pulse pressure (but little or no effect on diastolic pressure), and no net effect on peripheral resistance. Dopamine agonists (for example, fenoldopam) are presently being evaluated as potential antihypertensive agents. Some early studies with agonists acting at dopamine 1 and dopamine 2 receptors have shown blood pressure lowering in animals and hypertensive patients. See also *Catecholamines and hypertension*

Dopamine β-hydroxylase

Dopamine β-hydroxylase
Enzyme which catalyzes the hydroxylation of dopamine to noradrenaline (Figure 10). It is located in the storage vesicles.

Dopaminergic
Stimulated by, employing, or secreting dopamine. See also *Central catecholamines: Dopamine*

DOPEG
see *3,4-Dihydroxyphenylethylene glycol*

DOPGAL
see *3,4-Dihydroxyphenylglycolaldehyde*

Drug-induced hypertension
Hypertension may be caused or worsened by a variety of drugs either prescribed for another condition or purchased 'over the counter' in a pharmacy.
Glucocorticoids used orally or topically may, in excessive dosage, cause various features of Cushing's syndrome including hypertension. Mineralocorticoids in excessive doses, for example, 9 α-fludrocortisone used in the treatment of orthostatic hypotension, may also cause hypertension. Mineralocorticoid hypertension is also seen with carbenoxolone as well as in chronic excessive liquorice ingestion. It is well known that hypertension occurs in some patients taking the oral contraceptive pill and other oestrogen-containing preparations. Patients taking inhibitors of monoamine oxidase are at the risk of severe hypertension not only with ingestion of foods rich in tyramine (for example, cheese, Bovril), but also should avoid alpha-methyldopa and proprietary cold cures containing, for example, phenylpropanolamine. Finally, there are many drugs which are reported anecdotally to have caused hypertension, either alone or in combination with another agent.

Drug-induced lupus
A variety of drugs, including hydralazine

(and possibly alpha-methyldopa), may cause a syndrome similar to systemic lupus erythematosus.
Manifestations may vary from positive serology alone at one end of the spectrum to the full-blown picture of fever, arthritis, polyserositis, and haematological manifestations at the other end of the spectrum. Cerebral and renal manifestations are uncommon. Less than 10% of patients taking hydralazine develop drug-induced lupus which usually occurs after more than two months taking doses of 200 mg daily or more, although it can occur with lower doses. Drug-induced lupus usually disappears within six months of drug withdrawal. It is more common in women who are slow acetylators of the drug.
In some populations, hydralazine-induced lupus is associated with the tissue type HLA-DR4. In drug-induced lupus antinuclear factor testing is positive, but complement levels are generally normal and antibodies to native double-stranded DNA (common in spontaneous lupus) are very rarely found. See also *Alpha-methyldopa: Antinuclear factor: Hydralazine*

Dynorphins
These are opioid peptides found in the central nervous system. Both Dynorphin A and Dynorphin B are derived from the precursor peptide Prodynorphin. See also *Brain peptides and blood pressure control*

Dysarteriotony
Abnormality of blood pressure.

Dysplasias of renal arteries
see *Fibromuscular dysplasia*

E

Echocardiogram

(*also known as* Cardiac ultrasound)
Graphical record of the position, motion
and dimensions of the heart walls and
internal structures obtained by the use
of beams of ultrasonic waves directed
through the chest wall. Echocardiograms
provide a useful measure of ventricular
hypertrophy in hypertensive patients.
(See Figure 27c)

Eclampsia

Seizures which occur in a pregnant or
puerperal woman affected by pre-
eclampsia. Impending eclampsia is
suggested by the presence of headache,
blurred vision, nausea, epigastric pain,
hyper-reflexia and a rapid rise in blood
pressure. Management includes avoidance
of noise, sedation (for example, with
intravenous chlormethiazole), control of
blood pressure (for example, with
intravenous hydralazine), and induction
of labour. Eclampsia is one of the most
important causes of maternal death.
See also *Pregnancy and hypertension*

Ectopic ACTH secretion

Production of ACTH by tumours of
organs other than the anterior pituitary
gland. Ectopic ACTH secretion may cause
Cushing's syndrome.

Ectopic primary reninism

The clinical and biochemical changes
accompanying secretion of renin by
tumours not derived from tissue that
normally secretes it. This would,
therefore, exclude renin secretion by
juxtaglomerular renal tumours but include
secretion by other renal tumours and
extrarenal tumours. The syndrome
includes increased plasma renin activity,
secondary aldosteronism, and hypertension. The biochemical features, and
sometimes the hypertension, are cured by
removal of the responsible tumour if this is
possible. See *Renin*

Eicosanoid

Generic term for the prostaglandins,
leukotrienes and related compounds
derived from eicosatrienoic, eicosatetraenoic and eicosapentaenoic acids.
See also *Leukotrienes: Prostaglandins*

Eicosapentaenoic acid

One of the 20 carbon essential fatty
acid precursors of the prostaglandins,
leukotrienes and related compounds.
Eicosapentaenoic acid has five double
bonds (at positions 5, 8, 11, 14 and 17). See
also *Leukotrienes: Prostaglandins*

Eicosatetraenoic acid

Synonym for arachidonic acid. A 20
carbon fatty acid with four double bonds
at positions 5, 8, 11 and 14. See also
*Arachidonic acid: Leukotrienes:
Prostaglandins*

Eicosatetraynoic acid (ETYA)

Compound related to arachidonic acid
(eicosatetraenoic acid) which inhibits
transformation of the latter by either
the lipoxygenase or cyclo-oxygenase
pathways. See also *Arachidonic acid:
Cyclo-oxygenase: Leukotrienes:
Lipoxygenases: Prostaglandins*

Eicosatrienoic acid

Dihomo-γ-linolenic acid. A 20 carbon
essential fatty acid precursor of the
prostaglandins and related compounds,
which has three double bonds at positions
8, 11 and 14. See also *Leukotrienes:
Prostaglandins*

Ejaculation

Process that involves emission (movement
of semen into the urethra) and ejaculation
proper (propulsion of semen out of the

Ejaculation

urethra at orgasm). Emission is stimulated by the sympathetic nervous system. Semen is propelled from the urethra by contraction of the bulbocavernosus muscle which is controlled by a spinal reflex. Delayed ejaculation or failure to ejaculate may be a side-effect of certain antihypertensive drugs, especially those that interfere with the sympathetic nervous system, for example, adrenergic neurone blocking agents and ganglion blockers. Problems with ejaculation in a patient receiving an antihypertensive drug may, however, be unrelated to his medication. It may, nevertheless, be worth switching to an alternative drug to see if improvement results. See also *Adrenergic neurone blocking agents: Ganglion blocking drugs: Impotence*

Elastin

A glycoprotein which is the main constituent of the elastic fibres found, for example, in the tunica media of the arterial wall. Elastic fibres give the ability to recoil after transient stretch. Elastin molecules are joined together by covalent bands forming a cross-linked network.

Elderly and hypertension

(special contribution from Professor A. Amery, Universitaire Ziekenhuizen, Leuven, Belgium)
High blood pressure is frequent in the elderly and an increase in life expectancy in many Western countries has meant that hypertension has become important in this section of the population.
Furthermore among the several risk factors for cardiovascular disease, high blood pressure and especially systolic hypertension remains an important independent risk factor in the elderly population. However, such correlations do not prove *per se* a causal relationship between the hypertension and the cardiovascular complications.
Many clinicians were not convinced that lowering this high pressure by artificial means, such as hypotensive drugs, would decrease morbidity and mortality while preserving the quality of life of elderly patients. Therefore, intervention trials were undertaken which specifically tested the hypothesis that antihypertensive drug treatment would, in elderly hypertensive patients, lead to a decrease in morbidity and mortality. They included double-blind trials such as the Japanese trial (1981), the European trial in 1985 and 1986 and open but well-randomized trials, performed in general practice, for example, Coope's Study of Hypertension in the Elderly in 1986.

In addition elderly hypertensives were included in several other intervention trials in hypertensive patients and in some of them the results were presented separately for those patients above the age of 60 years; the latter were the Veterans Cooperative Studies (1972), the study on stroke survivors, Hypertension-Stroke Cooperators Study Group: effect of antihypertensive treatment on stroke recurrence (1974), the Hypertension Detection and Follow-up Program (1979) and the Australian Therapeutic Trial in Mild Hypertension (1981). By using meta-analysis Staessen *et al* in 1987 pooled the data related to the elderly of these various trials and showed a decrease in cardiovascular mortality (-28%, p = 0.016), and a decrease in cerebrovascular mortality (-41%, p = 0.030). The tendency to decrease was not significant for cardiac mortality (-24%, p = 0.126) or for mortality from ischaemic heart disease (-28%, p = 0.147) and fell just short of significance for mortality from all causes (-14%, p = 0.071). These data suggest that antihypertensive drug therapy may decrease mortality in the elderly, mainly by decreasing cerebrovascular accidents. In addition, combining all these trials non-fatal cardiovascular events were decreased on average by 50% (p < 0.001). Figure 47 illustrates such a decrease in cardiovascular study terminating events observed in the study of the European Working Party on High Blood Pressure in

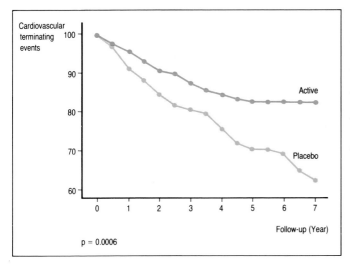

Cardiovascular
terminating
events

Active

Placebo

Follow-up (Year)

p = 0.0006

Cumulative percentage of
survivors without events
calculated for patients on
randomized treatment by
the life table method.
Cardiovascular
terminating events
include death and morbid
events.

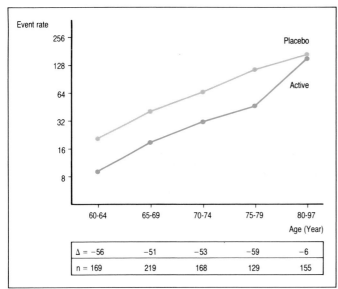

Event rate

Placebo

Active

| Δ = | −56 | −51 | −53 | −59 | −6 |
| n = | 169 | 219 | 168 | 129 | 155 |

Age (Year)

Figure 47b Elderly and
hypertension. Average
rates of cardiovascular
study terminating events
in the double-blind study
per 1000 patient 2 years.
Note the minimal
difference between
placebo and active
therapy in patients aged
80-97 years. Δ =
percentage reduction; n
= number of patients. The
event rate is presented on
a logarithmic scale.

the Elderly (EWPHE).
Although these data suggest that
hypotensive drug therapy may be
recommended in elderly hypertensive
patients, several areas of uncertainty
remain concerning the indications for drug
treatment. In most studies no patients
above the age of 80 years were admitted,
although in the EWPHE study, where
patients were admitted up to the age of
97 years, no decrease in events could be
shown in these very old patients (Figure
47). Thus, we would not recommend
antihypertensive drug treatment in very
elderly subjects on the basis of high
blood pressure *per se*, but only when

symptoms or signs are present which may be improved by treatment such as congestive heart failure, angina pectoris, or hypertensive encephalopathy.

It should be noted, also, that most of the reported studies did not admit patients with isolated systolic hypertension, but several intervention trials on this topic are now in planning or progress. Therefore, at present in patients with isolated systolic hypertension we would recommend hypotensive drug treatment only when signs or symptoms are present that are likely to be improved by treatment.

In the symptomless hypertensive patients below the age of 80 years the guidelines of the WHO-ISH (World Health Organization International Society of Hypertension) Committee recommend hypotensive drug treatment when, after applying general hygienic measures, the diastolic blood pressure remains above 100 mmHg after a three-month follow-up and 95 mmHg or above after a six-month follow-up period. See also *Coope's Study of Hypertension in the Elderly: European Working Party on High Blood Pressure in the Elderly Study: Multicentre studies of clinical outcome*

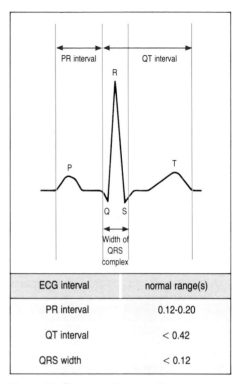

ECG interval	normal range(s)
PR interval	0.12-0.20
QT interval	< 0.42
QRS width	< 0.12

Figure 48 Electrocardiogram. Components of the electrocardiogram (ECG). The P-wave represents depolarization of the atria and the QRS complex represents depolarization of the ventricles. The T-wave results from repolarization of the ventricles. Normal ranges for various ECG intervals are shown in second(s). On an ECG tracing running at 25 mm/s one large square represents 0.2s and one small square 0.04s.

Electrocardiogram (ECG)
A graphical record of the variations in electrical potential recorded at the body surface associated with depolarization and repolarization of the muscle of the chambers of the heart (see Figure 48). Myocardial ischaemia and abnormalities of cardiac rhythm can be recognized readily. In the context of hypertension, the ECG is of most use as a measure of left ventricular hypertrophy. (Figure 27) See also *Cardiac hypertrophy: Exercise test: Left ventricular strain*

Electrolytes
see *Blood screening tests: Hypokalaemia*

Eledoisin
An endecapeptide produced in the salivary gland of a species of octopus. It is the precursor of a group of biologically

active peptides and has vasodilator and hypotensive properties.

Embolus
Clot or other foreign body brought by the blood stream from another vessel or the heart and lodging in a smaller vessel, occluding the blood supply to areas distal to the obstruction. See also *Cerebral infarction*

Enalapril
An angiotensin I converting enzyme inhibitor.

Encephalins
A pair of opioid peptides. Methionine (met-) encephalin is derived from processing of proencephalin. Leucine (leu-) encephalin is produced from both proencephalin and prodynorphin. See also *Brain peptides and blood pressure control*

Endarterectomy
Surgical removal of the atheromatous tunica intima of an artery.
Sometimes, particularly in the United States, the technique is used to treat carotid artery atherosclerosis. Although remarkable improvement in the symptoms of individual patients may result, evidence that the technique is superior to treatment with antiplatelet agents, for example, aspirin, for the majority of patients with transient ischaemic attacks is not strong.

Endarteritis obliterans
see *Arteriosclerosis obliterans*

Endocrine hypertension
Hypertension secondary to disease of one of the endocrine glands. Probably less than 1% of cases of hypertension have an endocrine cause. Apart from adrenal disease hypertension may also be a feature of acromegaly, primary hyperparathyroidism, primary hypothyroidism, and thyrotoxicosis.

Endoplasmic reticulum
The system of branching membrane-bound cavities found in the cytoplasm of nearly all cells of higher plants and animals, which acts as a major intracellular store of calcium in non-muscle cells.

Endorphins
A family of opioid peptides which include beta-endorphin, derived from pro-opiomelanocortin, and alpha- and beta-neoendorphins, derived from prodyn-

orphin. See also *Brain peptides and blood pressure control: Encephalins: Opioid peptides*

Endothelium
The layer of epithelial cells lining the blood and lymphatic vessels as well as the cavity of the heart.

Endralazine (Endrallazine)
A vasodilator which is chemically related to hydralazine, but has a longer duration of action and may not cause drug-induced lupus. Limited data suggest that the drug needs to be given twice daily. See also *Hydralazine: Drug-induced Lupus*

Enteramine
Synonym (little used) for 5-hydroxy-tryptamine.

Environment and hypertension
Certain features of an individual's way of life and surroundings may influence the risk of developing hypertension. For example, physical work, diet and obesity, alcohol consumption, use of the oral contraceptive pill, pregnancy, and psychosocial stress. See also *Alcohol: Central nervous system and hypertension: Contraceptive pill: Diet and hypertension: Ethnic differences in hypertension: Exercise: Heredity and hypertension: Obesity and hypertension: Pregnancy and hypertension: Stress and hypertension*

Ephedrine
A sympathomimetic drug with central and peripheral effects. It stimulates both alpha- and beta-adrenergic receptors. The peripheral effects are caused partly by stimulating release of noradrenaline. Ephedrine raises systolic and usually also diastolic blood pressure, partly due to vasoconstriction, but mainly due to cardiac stimulation. Now mainly used as a nasal decongestant, but was used as a bronchodilator before specific beta$_2$-agonists became available.

Epinephrectomy
Synonym for adrenalectomy

Epinephrine
Synonym for adrenaline.
Aldrich (1901) used the term after the work on "epinephrin" by Abel in the same year. The term "adrenaline" derives from Takamine's description of the active principle of the suprarenal (adrenal) gland in 1901. See also *Noradrenaline (norepinephrine)*

Epistaxis
A nose bleed. Some studies have found a higher frequency of hypertension than would have been expected by chance in patients with epistaxis which had no local cause. Epistaxis, however, is not a frequent feature in patients with high blood pressure. In patients with epistaxis who are hypertensive, lowering of blood pressure often helps to control the bleeding. It should be remembered, however, that the blood pressure of patients who have elevated levels at the time of an epistaxis may subsequently settle to normal levels.

Epithiazide
A thiazide diuretic.

1,2-Epoxy-3(p-nitrophenoxy)propane
An aspartyl protease inhibitor which has powerful inhibitory effects on renin. See also *Aspartyl proteases: Renin*

Ergotamine
An alkaloid drug used in the treatment of migraine.
Ergotamine has complex cardiovascular effects, producing constriction of both arteries and veins. Effects are probably mediated by interactions with alpha-adrenergic receptors, tryptaminergic receptors, or both. Dihydroergotamine has been used in the treatment of orthostatic hypotension because its vasoconstrictor activity affects capacitance vessels (the venous side of the circulation) more than resistance vessels. See also *Dihydro-ergotamine: Orthostatic hypotension*

Erythrocyte ion transport systems
The red blood cell has a number of membrane-bound proteins responsible for transporting ions across the cell membrane. Since such mechanisms may be common to different cell types the erythrocyte, because of its easy availability, has been used to compare intracellular ion concentrations and the activities of these ion transport systems in cells from normal subjects and patients with essential hypertension. See also *Cell sodium hypothesis: Intracellular cations in essential hypertension: Ion transport systems*

Erythropoietin
A circulating glycoprotein produced largely in the kidneys (probably by epithelial cells in the glomeruli) but also, in humans, in some other organs, particularly the liver. Its production is stimulated by hypoxia or anaemia. It stimulates production of red blood cells by causing certain precursor (stem) cells in the bone marrow to differentiate. There is an association between erythrocytosis (increased red blood cell mass) caused by inappropriate erythropoietin production and renal cysts, renal carcinoma, as well as hydronephrosis. In some of these cases there is also hypertension. See also *Hydronephrosis: Polycythaemia*

Essential hypertension
(special contribution from Dr A.F. Lever, MRC Blood Pressure Unit, Western Infirmary, Glasgow, Scotland)
Definition, diagnosis and decision on treatment
Essential hypertension is an important but ill-defined condition. Its importance lies in the close and positive relation between blood pressure and the risk of subsequent development of stroke, coronary disease

and renal and cardiac failure. The condition is common, and is characterized by high blood pressure of unknown cause, known causes of hypertension such as Conn's syndrome and renal artery disease having been excluded before the diagnosis is reached.

The indefinable quality of essential hypertension is illustrated by an interesting but unresolved controversy, which Sir George Pickering and Sir Robert (later Lord) Platt debated between the 1940s and 1960s.

According to Pickering high blood pressure cannot be defined as an entity separable qualitatively from normal in the sense that patients with pernicious anaemia are qualitatively different from normal. Nor can it be separated quantitatively since, as illustrated in Figure 49, there is no dip in the frequency distribution of blood pressure separating patients with and without essential hypertension. There is, therefore, no diagnostic borderline between normal and abnormally high blood pressure. According to Platt, essential hypertension is a disease qualitatively separable from normal in the sense that individuals have or have not the gene for the condition. Pickering challenged Platt's epidemiological evidence but neither doubted the existence of an important genetic component. The controversy subsided unresolved, probably because both protagonists were partly correct.

In practice, clinicians and investigators may not need to define hypertension. Their need is to establish the level of blood pressure above which treatment by hypotensive drugs does more good than harm. By implication there may be a level below this point where risk from increased pressure still exists, but where hypotensive treatment is either neutral or harmful in its net effect. An important dilemma for the physician arising from this is illustrated schematically in Figure 49. In this figure the frequency distribution of blood pressure for individuals in a large general population in the upper panel shows the familiar bell-shaped curve skewed to the right. In three arbitrary categories from the right are 'severe', 'moderate' and 'mild' hypertension. The diagnoses here are usually based on several measurements in the untreated state, but as blood pressure tends to fall when serial measurements are made, mild hypertension in one study may differ from mild hypertension in another. The risks to the individual are shown in the second panel. These are graded in relation to arterial pressure. The gradient for stroke is steeper than that for coronary disease, but the second is commoner and, therefore, more individuals are at risk from coronary disease.

The third panel illustrates the problem as seen by the community physician. Although overall risk in an individual with mild hypertension is less than that in a moderate or severe hypertensive, 'attributable' risk (risk to individual × numbers at risk) is higher in mild hypertension because there are more individuals at risk. More heart attacks and strokes are to be expected in mild than severe hypertensives therefore.

The dilemma is illustrated in the fourth panel. Knowing that mild hypertensives are at risk, that hypotensive drugs lower blood pressure usually without side-effects, and that trials have shown benefit from treatment in moderate hypertension, the physician will be tempted to treat mild hypertensives. Recent evidence gives some idea of the benefit to be expected. The risk of stroke will be reduced by approximately 50% but in absolute terms this is not so impressive. To save one stroke about 50 mild hypertensives will need treatment for 10 years. Set against this undoubted benefit is the cost, inconvenience and likelihood of developing a minor side-effect. A cost-benefit analysis of such varied data is difficult to judge scientifically or clinically. It may also be that within the wide span of mild hypertension some groups will be shown to benefit

Essential hypertension

more than others in which case treatment could be concentrated on those expected to benefit most.

Pathogenesis

Although the cause of essential hypertension is not known there are some interesting clues. The genetic component is beyond question and yet serial measurements by Miall and colleagues in South Wales show that blood pressure rises very slowly, even in essential hypertensives, by a few mmHg per year usually. Thus, although patients may be born with the disease, it is expressed genetically not as a difference from normal at the outset in infancy but as a rate of rise of pressure which is steeper than normal in adult life. These observations restrict the number of plausible explanations for pathogenesis. Almost all the candidate mechanisms are quick-acting: excess steroids, abnormal body sodium, increased dietary sodium, increased catecholamines or sympathetic nerve activity and many others; all exert their pressor effect quickly (varying in their speed of action from a few seconds to a few days). If a genetically-determined abnormality of one of these mechanisms is by itself the primary cause of essential hypertension, it must be

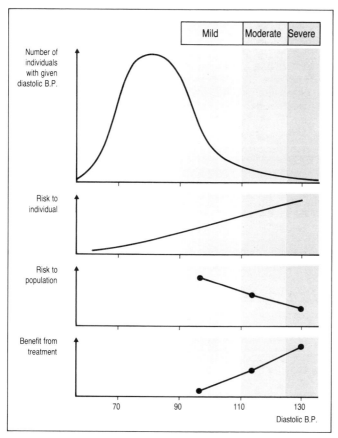

Figure 49 Essential hypertension. Blood pressure is distributed unimodally (top section): thus there are more patients with mild hypertension than with moderate or severe hypertension. On the other hand, individual risk is positively correlated with blood pressure (section 2) so that severer degrees of hypertension are associated with higher individual risk. However, because of the numerical preponderance of mildly hypertensive patients the number of individuals at risk in the population is much greater for mild than for moderate or severe hypertension (section 3). The greatest population benefit, therefore, comes from measures directed at the mildest degrees of hypertension whilst the greatest individual benefit accrues from treating patients with moderate and severe hypertension (section 4).

expressed slowly and yet in sufficient degree to explain the hypertension at all stages by its quick-acting property. None of the candidate mechanisms has this pattern of derangement. An alternative suggested by Folkow and others is that a double mechanism is at work, that the primary cause of essential hypertension is a minor abnormality in a quick-acting mechanism which is slowly amplified by a second positive feed-back process involving vascular hypertrophy. See also *Folkow's theory: Vascular hypertrophy in hypertension*

Ethacrynic acid
A loop diuretic which is less commonly used than frusemide, partly because of gastrointestinal intolerance. Development of deafness, which has rarely been permanent, is a serious but rare complication of treatment with ethacrynic acid. Transient deafness has also been reported with frusemide and bumetanide. See also *Diuretics: Loop diuretics*

Ethinyl oestradiol
An oestrogen which is a common constituent of the combined oral contraceptive. See *Contraceptive pill*

Ethnic differences in hypertension
(special contribution from Professor Norman M. Kaplan, The University of Texas, Dallas, Texas, U.S.A.)
Blacks suffer from hypertension more than whites and this results in more morbidity and mortality from strokes and renal damage in blacks. More limited data suggest that Asians and Hispanics tend to be intermediate between whites and blacks in their prevalence of hypertension.
Before the age of 20, whites and blacks have similar levels of blood pressure but, thereafter, levels tend to be higher in blacks. In some comparisons such as among factory workers in Birmingham, England, mean levels of blood pressure are similar among the different ethnic groups but hypertension is more frequent among blacks and Asians than among whites. Numerous environmental differences, in addition to genetic susceptibility, have been proposed to explain the higher prevalence and severity of hypertension in blacks. These include, more obesity, particularly in black women, higher dietary sodium and less dietary potassium intakes, and lower socioeconomical and educational status with less access to health care and treatment. Pathophysiological differences have been observed which may reflect these environmental differences, including higher body fluid volume, reduced excretion of a sodium load, lower levels of plasma renin activity, enhanced vascular responses to mental stress, and a smaller responsiveness to beta-blocker therapy. Some investigators find a higher intracellular sodium concentration within red blood cells along with reduced red blood cell sodium-potassium adenosine triphosphatase activity in both normotensive and hypertensive blacks than in whites.
Using these various findings, an explanation for the higher prevalence of hypertension in blacks can be constructed, based upon a genetic defect in sodium excretion that is more prevalent among blacks. Perhaps blacks, who originally lived in hot, arid climates wherein sodium conservation was important for survival, evolved the physiological machinery which protects them in their original habitat, but makes it difficult for them to handle the excessive sodium they ingest when they migrate. Among a number of studies which support this view is one comparing tribal and urban Xhosa people of Southern Africa: those who migrated had higher blood pressures which rose progressively with age, whereas in the tribal group, pressures were low and rose very little with age. Only two of many factors examined were related to the

Ethnic differences in hypertension

rising pressure in the urban blacks: increased dietary sodium and increased body weight.

When hypertensive, blacks suffer more strokes, cardiac enlargement, and renal damage but have the same susceptibility to coronary heart disease as do whites. This may reflect, on the one hand, barriers to health care which reduce the control of their hypertension but, on the other hand, a tendency to lower levels of serum cholesterol and high levels of high density lipoprotein-cholesterol among blacks. Moreover, when these barriers have been removed, as in the Hypertension Detection and Follow-up Program in the United States, the rate of achievement of the goal of therapy was slower for blacks than whites. With continued therapy, however, blacks achieved the greatest reduction in mortality. See also *Cell sodium hypothesis: Ion transport systems*

Ethylene-diamine-tetra-acetic acid (EDTA)

Chelating agents such as EDTA can be used to inhibit angiotensin I converting enzyme in plasma probably by binding either Ca^{2+} or Zn^{2+} which are considered essential for the function of the enzyme. Renal clearance of ^{51}Cr-EDTA is also used as a measure of glomerular filtration rate. See also *Creatine clearance: Glomerular filtration rate*

European Working Party on High Blood Pressure in the Elderly (EWPHE) study (Lancet (1985) 1:1349-1354)

A double-blind, randomized, placebo-controlled trial of antihypertensive treatment in 840 patients aged 60 years or more (average age 72 years). The trial included patients with both sitting diastolic blood pressure on placebo of 90-119 mmHg and systolic pressure in the range 160-239 mmHg. The patients were randomized to placebo or active treatment (hydrochlorothiazide and triamterene). If blood pressure remained raised, alpha-methyldopa was added to the active regime and matched placebo was added in the placebo group. 'Intention-to-treat' analysis showed a non-significant change in total mortality with treatment but cardiovascular mortality was significantly reduced.

Interestingly, this included a significant decrease in cardiac deaths as well as an insignificant decrease in cerebrovascular mortality.

The trial showed a substantial reduction in deaths from myocardial infarction (-60%, $p = 0.043$) although non-fatal myocardial infarction tended to be more frequent in the active treatment group. Non-terminating cerebrovascular events were also reduced (-52%, $p = 0.026$). Benefits of treatment were offset to some degree by decreased glucose tolerance and increased serum concentrations of uric acid and creatinine in the actively treated group. See also *Coope's Study of Hypertension in the Elderly: Elderly and hypertension: Multicentre studies of clinical outcome*

Evans blue dye

(Herbert Meleon Evans, U.S. anatomist and embryologist, 1882-1971)

A dye which binds to plasma proteins. Used in the measurement of plasma volume. See also *Blood volume*

Exchangeable sodium and potassium

Exchangeable sodium (Na_E) or potassium (K_E) is that fraction of the total body content of those ions which will equilibrate with exogenously administered isotopes (^{24}Na and ^{43}K). The difference between total body sodium and exchangeable sodium probably represents the large pool of non-exchangeable sodium in bone. Mean values for Na_E and K_E are normal in untreated essential hypertension. In contrast to normotensive subjects, however, in essential hypertension Na_E appears to be positively related to both systolic and diastolic pressure. See also *Body sodium and potassium*

Excitation-contraction coupling

The process by which depolarization of the muscle fibre membrane initiates contraction. Depolarization causes an increase in intracellular calcium concentration. Calcium then binds to calmodulin in smooth muscle or troponin C in skeletal and cardiac muscle. The protein then undergoes a conformational change and interacts with the contractile apparatus. See also *Calcium: Calmodulin: Troponin C*

Excretory urography

see *Intravenous pyelography*

Exercise

Physical exertion. Evidence is accumulating to suggest that moderate regular exercise may have a blood pressure lowering effect independent of the changes in dietary habits, lifestyle and weight loss often associated with taking up exercise. Exercise should be encouraged particularly in obese hypertensive patients as it should make weight reduction easier to achieve. Exercise is also associated with an increase in high density lipoprotein cholesterol levels and this may be associated with a reduced risk of atherosclerotic complications. See also *Isometric exercise: Isotonic exercise*

Exercise test

The recording of the electrocardiogram during exercise is often useful in the diagnosis of angina, particularly when the pain is not typical and / or the resting electrocardiogram is normal or nearly normal. Depression of the ST segment is one of the most significant changes occurring with exercise. In hypertensive patients with left ventricular hypertrophy a 'strain' pattern may develop with exercise giving a false impression of myocardial ischaemia secondary to coronary artery disease. See also *Cardiac hypertrophy: Left ventricular strain*

Extracellular fluid volume (ECFV)

About 20% of total body fluid is extracellular (this includes plasma and interstitial fluid). It is difficult to measure, but is best estimated using radioactively labelled inulin. Most workers have found normal values for ECFV in essential hypertension. See also *Blood volume: Inulin clearance*

Extrasystole

A premature cardiac contraction that is independent of the normal rhythm and is caused by an impulse arising in a part of the heart other than the sinoatrial node. More common in hypertensive patients who have left ventricular hypertrophy. A ventricular rather than atrial origin is regarded generally of more adverse prognostic significance. See also *Cardiac hypertrophy*

F

Fabry's disease (angiokeratoma corporis diffusum)
(Johannes Fabry, German dermatologist, 1860-1930)
A rare X-linked inborn error of glycosphingolipid metabolism fully manifested in hemizygous males, and may also be partially manifested in heterozygous females.
Fabry's disease is due to deficiency of alpha-galactosidase A, causing abnormal deposition of glycosphingolipid. Clinical features include telangiectasia which may lead to diagnosis in childhood. Other features include diminished sweating, acral pain (leading to confusion with Still's disease), paraesthesiae and corneal opacities. It may cause myocardial infarction or congestive cardiac failure. Hypertension may develop due to involvement of renal parenchymal vessels. Renal failure is common in the second to fourth decades of life. Fabry's disease is diagnosed by showing decreased enzyme activity in many tissues. Treatment is at present purely symptomatic.

Faintness
Term used to denote vague dizziness or light-headedness. May precede syncope.
See also *Giddiness: Syncope*

Familial combined hyperlipidaemia
Familial combined hyperlipidaemia can occur with hypertriglyceridaemia alone, with hypercholesterolaemia alone, or with raised plasma levels of both lipids. Differentiation between familial hypertriglyceridaemia and familial combined hyperlipidaemia as a cause of isolated hypertriglyceridaemia is difficult but important, as only those with the combined disorder appear to be at increased risk of atherosclerosis. Hypertriglyceridaemic patients with a family history of ischaemic heart disease

are more likely to have combined hyperlipidaemia. An entirely negative family history would make one less inclined to treat hypertriglyceridaemia aggressively in an attempt to reduce the risk of ischaemic heart disease. See also *Atherosclerosis: Cholesterol: Familial hypercholesterolaemia: Familial hypertriglyceridaemia: Familial hyperlipoproteinaemia: Lipoproteins: Triglyceride*

Familial hyperlipoproteinaemia
Increased fasting plasma concentrations of lipoproteins associated with raised levels of cholesterol and / or triglyceride may have a familial basis.
Familial hypercholesterolaemia is associated with a greatly increased risk of atherosclerosis, but familial hyper-triglyceridaemia does not appear to be an important risk factor for atheroma. Familial combined hyperlipidaemia is, however, associated with an increased risk of atherosclerosis. See also *Cholesterol: Familial combined hyperlipidaemia: Lipoproteins: Triglyceride*

Familial hypercholesterolaemia
A monogenic, dominantly inherited disorder associated with raised levels of low density lipoprotein (LDL) cholesterol caused by a group of defects in the function of the LDL receptor.
Patients develop skin and / or tendon xanthomata and may have a corneal arcus before the age of 40 years. About 5% of male heterozygotes have had their first episode of ischaemic heart disease by age 30 years. Females seem to be affected later. Treatment is by diet and the use of drugs such as cholestyramine. It would seem wise to treat vigorously coexistent hypertension. See also *Cholesterol: Familial hyperlipoproteinaemia: Lipoproteins: Low density lipoprotein*

Familial hypertension
see *Family history: Heredity and hypertension*

Familial hypertriglyceridaemia
Raised fasting plasma concentration of triglyceride is due to overproduction of very low density lipoprotein (VLDL) in two distinct familial disorders: familial hypertriglyceridaemia and familial combined hyperlipidaemia.

Other rare causes of inherited hypertriglyceridaemia include primary lipoprotein lipase deficiency. Severe hypertriglyceridaemia (for example, plasma triglyceride concentration of 20 mmol / l) may lead to saturation of lipoprotein lipase and impaired removal of chylomicrons. Eruptive xanthomata, lipaemia retinalis and acute pancreatitis may result. For treatment see *Triglyceride*. See also *Cholesterol: Familial hyperlipoproteinaemia: Lipoproteins*

Family history
Patients with essential hypertension often give a history of hypertension or premature vascular disease (ischaemic heart disease or cerebrovascular accident) in parents, grandparents, siblings or other relatives. There may also be a family history of renal failure. Patients with secondary hypertension may also give a positive family history, for example, polycystic kidneys, phaeochromocytoma, and primary hyperparathyroidism. See also *Essential hypertension: Heredity and hypertension: Secondary hypertension*

Fatty streaks
Fatty streaks are found in the intima and are thought to represent the early precursors of the atheromatous plaques in the arteries of patients with atherosclerosis.

The streaks are flat lesions which are lipid-rich and contain mainly macrophages but also smooth muscle cells. They are commonly found in children and young adults at sites similar to those where plaques of atheroma are found in later life. In experimental animals diet-induced hypercholesterolaemia leads to changes in the endothelium and in the monocytes of the blood causing increased monocyte adherence, subendothelial migration, accumulation of lipid to form foam cells, and slow accumulation of smooth muscle cells to form fatty streaks. A similar process may occur in man, explaining the mechanism by which patients with hypercholesterolaemia are predisposed to atherosclerosis. See also *Atherosclerosis: Cholesterol*

Felodipine
A calcium entry blocker of the dihydropyridine class. Properties are similar to nifedipine. See *Calcium antagonists*

Fibre, accelerating / accelerator
Adrenergic neurones transmitting the impulses which stimulate an increase in heart rate. See also *Cardiac rate: Sympathetic nervous system*

Fibre, depressor
When applied to the heart, refers to vagal nerve fibres which when activated cause a decrease in heart rate. May also be applied to nerve fibre, activation of which causes vasodilatation. See also *Parasympathetic nervous system: Vagus nerve*

Fibre, pressor
Noradrenergic nerve fibres supplying the arterioles, activation of which leads to vasoconstriction and an increase in blood pressure. See also *Fibre, vasodilator: Sympathetic nervous system*

Fibre, vasodilator
Cholinergic nerve fibres accompanying the sympathetic nerves supplying the resistance vessels of skeletal muscle. Activation of these cholinergic fibres leads to vasodilatation.

Fibre, vasomotor
Nerve fibres supplying mainly the arterioles, activation of which causes vasoconstriction or vasodilatation.
See *Fibre, pressor: Fibre, vasodilator*

Fibrillation, atrial
An abnormality of cardiac rhythm characterized clinically by a pulse which is irregular in rhythm and volume.
The electrocardiogram (Figure 50) shows absence of P-waves and irregular QRS complexes. May be found most commonly in mitral valve disease, thyrotoxicosis and in ischaemic heart disease, which may be associated with hypertension. Patients in atrial fibrillation are at increased risk of cerebrovascular accident compared with patients in sinus rhythm, presumably

due to cerebral embolism. The use of anticoagulants (for example, warfarin) in an attempt to prevent embolism in patients with atrial fibrillation, but without mitral valve disease, has not been justified by controlled trials but is a practice widely adopted. The ventricular rate in atrial fibrillation can be controlled with digoxin.

Fibrillation, ventricular
An abnormality of cardiac rhythm which is the commonest immediate cause of sudden death. It presents clinically as a cardiac arrest.
The electrocardiogram shows broad, bizarre, irregular complexes. Ventricular fibrillation is most commonly due to myocardial infarction, which is more common in hypertensive patients. Treatment is by means of DC defibrillation and the remainder of the standard management of cardiac arrest.

Fibrin
The insoluble protein formed in the blood clotting process from plasma fibrinogen. Studies have shown that fibrin is found in increasing amounts with ageing in the intima of large arteries. In areas of cholesterol deposition there is often an overlying layer of fibrin. See also *Arterial wall: Atherosclerosis: Fibrinoid arteriolar necrosis*

Fibrinoid arteriolar necrosis
A pathological change found in the arterioles of, for example, the kidney and brain, of patients with malignant phase hypertension. Fibrinoid necrosis is usually superimposed on arteriolar hyalinosis. Areas of necrosis appear histologically as granular, eosinophilic zones with indefinite borders against the pink background of hyalin. These zones seem to contain fibrin which may be derived from plasma fibrinogen. The increased permeability of the blood vessel wall in severe hypertension may allow fibrin to be deposited within the wall. In the brain, both lacunar infarction and cerebral

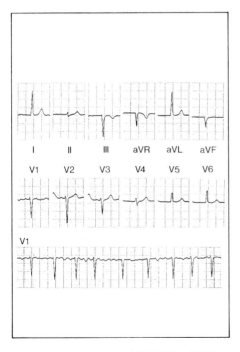

Figure 50 Fibrillation, atrial. A 12 lead ECG showing atrial fibrillation, the ventricular rate is irregular and atrial fibrillation activity is clearly seen on lead V_1.

haemorrhage in hypertensive patients have been shown to be associated with fibrinoid necrosis in the surrounding arterioles. See *Hyalin: Malignant phase hypertension*

Fibromuscular dysplasia
A heterogenous group of lesions in which fibrous or fibromuscular thickening may involve the intima, media or, rarely, the adventitia of, for example, the renal arteries.
Fibromuscular dysplasia may cause renal artery stenosis, although atherosclerosis is a much commoner cause. Patients with renal artery stenosis due to fibromuscular dysplasia tend to be younger than those in whom the stenosis is due to athero-sclerosis. In medial fibromuscular dysplasia (the largest group) women are more frequently affected than men. See also *Arterial wall: Intima: Intimal fibroplasia of renal artery: Media: Medial fibromuscular dysplasia of renal arteries: Renovascular hypertension*

Fick principle
(Adolphe Eugen Fick, German physiologist, 1829-1901)
The principle that the amount of a substance taken up by an organ (or the body) per unit time is given by multiplying the A-V difference (arterial minus venous concentration) by the blood flow.
Used to calculate cardiac output from knowledge of the oxygen consumed by the body and the A-V difference across the lungs. See also *Cardiac output*

Filtration fraction
The ratio of glomerular filtration rate (GFR) to renal plasma flow. The normal range is 0.16–0.20. Decreased systemic arterial pressure lowers GFR less than renal plasma flow and filtration fraction, therefore, rises in this situation. See also *Glomerular filtration rate: Renal plasma flow*

Fletcher factor
Synonym for plasma kallikrein named

from the family of the first patient. See also *Kallikreins*

Fludrocortisone
(9-alpha-fludrocortisone: 9-alpha-fluorohydrocortisone: 9-alpha-fluorocortisol) A very potent synthetic mineralocorticoid drug (two to three times more potent than aldosterone) used in the treatment of Addison's disease and orthostatic hypotension.
In Addison's disease adequacy of mineralocorticoid replacement can be gauged by measuring plasma renin activity, which should be brought down to normal with treatment. In excessive dosage, 9-alpha-fludrocortisone may cause hypertension. See also *Drug-induced hypertension: Mineralocorticoid activity: Mineralocorticoid-induced hypertension*

Fluorescein angiography
A technique for outlining the retinal vasculature using a fluorescent dye.
In patients with malignant phase hypertension there may be some debate as to the presence of papilloedema on ophthalmoscopy, though prognostically this problem is not important. Fluorescein angiography in malignant hypertension shows engorged vessels arising from the choroidal and retinal circulation and in late pictures there will be leakage of dye producing a fluorescent disc. Elsewhere in the fundi of these patients angiography will show areas of non-perfusion of the capillary bed and leakage of dye from the arteries. (Figure 51) See also *Hypertensive retinopathy*

Fluoroprednisolone
(9-alpha-Fluoroprednisolone)
A synthetic mineralocorticoid drug.
Cases of hypertension with this drug have been associated with its use as a topical agent. See also *Drug-induced hypertension: Mineralocorticoid activity: Mineralocorticoid-induced hypertension*

Folkow's theory

Folkow's theory (Folkow's hypothesis)

(B. Folkow, Swedish physician, born 1921)

Folkow's pioneering work on vascular hypertrophy emphasized the role of load-induced resistance vessel hypertrophy in producing vascular hyper-reactivity. Although hypertrophy is normally thought of as a consequence of hypertension it could play an important role in maintaining blood pressure in most forms of hypertension and in particular in essential hypertension in man.

According to this theory exaggerated pressor responses conditioned, for instance, by an overactive sympathetic nervous system give rise to resistance vessel hypertrophy and hyper-reactivity. As a consequence there is increased resistance for any given level of smooth muscle tone and blood pressure is therefore reset upwards. An interesting development of the theory is the suggestion that in genetically predisposed patients and animals the relationship between hypertrophy and pressure load is disturbed in favour of hypertrophy,

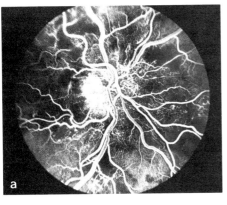
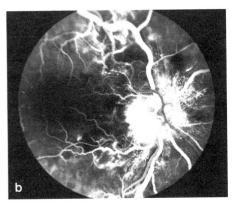
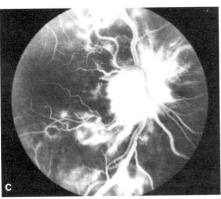
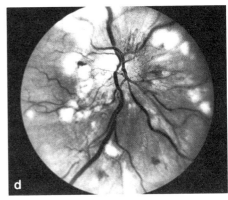

Figure 51 Fluorescein angiography.
Fluorescein angiogram obtained in a patient with malignant hypertension. Note the engorged vessels overlying the disc (51a)

and the persistence of dye which has leaked from the vessels (51b & 51c). Fig 51d shows micro-infarcts where perfusion has been blocked.

thereby predisposing to blood pressure elevation. See also *Vascular hypertrophy and hypertension*

Framingham Study
(Medical World Press: 1981 103-127).
A prospective longitudinal study of 5209 men and women selected by randomized sampling from the adult population (30-62 years old) of Framingham, Massachuetts, set up in 1949. The objective of the Framingham Study was to identify factors related to the development of cardiovascular disease and stroke. This carefully observed population has proved of major importance in supplementing data from cross-sectional studies. Thus the Framingham study has confirmed the positive association between blood pressure and weight, heart rate, alcohol consumption, glucose and haematocrit and the inverse association between blood pressure and smoking. It has also confirmed the importance of hypertension as a risk factor for cardiovascular mortality, but unlike insurance data, it also demonstrates the association between hypertension and cardiovascular morbidity (that is non-fatal heart attacks and strokes).
From the clinical viewpoint the Framingham study has shown that the risks of hypertension (expressed as absolute, relative or attributable risk) are as great in the elderly as in younger subjects. It has demonstrated the additive effects of other risk factors such as serum cholesterol, glucose intolerance, cigarette smoking or hypertrophy on the ECG for cardiovascular disease. It has also demonstrated the importance of systolic blood pressure which showed a slightly better association with cardiovascular disease than diastolic pressure.
The Framingham data was also used to demonstrate a relationship between some lipid sub-fractions and cardiovascular disease: this relationship was favourable for high density lipoproteins (HDL) and unfavourable for low density lipoproteins

(LDL). The Framingham study is essentially observational. It does not set out to analyse the effect of any particular intervention but the information gained from it provides the basis for more targetted studies of specific interventions.

Free water clearance (C_{H_2O})
The difference between the urine volume (V) and the osmolal clearance.

$$\text{Free water clearance} = V - \frac{U_{OSM}V}{P_{OSM}}$$

where U_{OSM} = urine osmolality and P_{OSM} = plasma osmolality.
From this it can be deduced that C_{H_2O} is zero when urine and plasma are isotonic, negative when urine is hypertonic and positive when urine is hypotonic. C_{H_2O} represents the amount of water (ml / min) that would have to be added to or subtracted from the urine voided in unit time to render the specimen isotonic with plasma. Measurements of free water clearance during maximal diuresis and in the same subjects under conditions of dehydration have been used to infer the intrarenal sites of action of diuretics.

Frusemide
(*also known as* Furosemide) A commonly used loop diuretic. Used, as are the other members of this group, in hypertension where renal function is impaired and also forms part of the standard treatment of cardiac failure. Common side-effects are abnormalities of fluid and electrolyte balance, particularly with excessive dosage. Hyperuricaemia is a common associated biochemical abnormality. Gastrointestinal intolerance is less common than with ethacrynic acid. Decreased glucose tolerance is rarer than with a thiazide. Rarer side-effects include marrow depression, hepatic dysfunction, interstitial nephritis, and transient deafness. See *Diuretics: Loop diuretics*

Furosemide
Synonym for frusemide.

Acknowledgements

We would like to thank the publishers for permission to reproduce
the following illustrations:

Figures 4 and 7 from G W Herd et al, Clinical Endocrinology
(1987) **26** 699–705

Figures 9,21, 36, 44a and 44b from Hypertension illustrated edited
by John Swales, 1982 (Gower Medical Publishing)

Table 1 from R J Lefkowitz et al, New England Journal of Medicine
(1984) **310**, 1570

Figure 34 and Table 2 from Handbook of hypertension edited by
W H Birkenhäger and J L Reid (1984) volume 1. Figure 45 from
volume 2 (Elsevier Science Publishers BV)

Table 5 from R H Grimm and D B Hunninghake, American Journal
of Medicine (1986) **80**, supplement 2a

Table 10 from P J M Sloan and D G Beevers, European Heart
Journal (1983) **4**, no 4 (Academic Press Ltd)

Table 14 from Fundamentals of clinical endocrinology by R Hall
(1980) chapter 20 (Churchill Livingstone)

Table 16 from D E Grobbee, Current Opinion in Cardiology (1986)
1, 607–613 (Gower Academic Journals)

Figure 10b from Review of medical physiolology edited by
W F Ganong, section 4, 12th edition 1985 (Lange Medical
Publications)

Figure 19 from D J Reis et al, Clinical and experimental hypertension (A) (1984) **6**, 221 (Marcel Dekker, Inc.)

Figure 47a from A Amery et al, Lancet (1985) **i**, 1349–1354
Figure 47b from A Amery et al, Lancet (1986) **ii**, 589–592

We are very grateful to Emanuel Rosen MD FRCS for the fluorescein angiograms in figure 51 and would also like to thank Dr
Brendan Hicks for the illustration of diabetic nephropathy in
figure 46.